PRAISE FOR AND *TO*

"Dementia, in its many forms, remains all too common in our world. *Touch the Spirit* is one of best books on staying connected to someone with dementia. Inspiring, clearly written and authoritative, this book is highly recommended."
~ Larry Dossey, M.D., author of *The Power of Premonitions and the One Mind*

"Deborah Forrest can teach you how to care for and be with a loved one with dementia. She knows the science and considers the mysterious and the spiritual. Plus, she writes as though she were having a conversation with you."
~Thomas Moore, Ph.D., author of *Care of the Soul*

"Deborah Forrest's *Touch the Spirit* is the most comprehensive, ground-breaking book on dementia I have every read. I lost my father 2 years ago to the disease and when I read "*the gift of profound dementia, especially the Alzheimer's type, is that nothing said to the person will be registered in the person's physical memory banks. It will be remembered in the soul's registry of life events*" I felt like it was a message from my father telling me that no moment had been wasted. Her deep understanding of the many forms of dementia will be of great value to the millions of people whose lives will be affected by this confounding disease."
~Catherine Oxenburg, Actress & CEO of Holy Cow Productions

"Deborah Forrest is not only a valuable Clinical Psychologist, nurse and lecturer, but a true humanist who is able to get her outstanding qualities of understanding the concepts of dementia, communication and the importance of the soul into a book that produces a needed resource of great human value. She is brave to help bridge the gap between dementia and the metaphysical heart, and how to understand their connection. She displays knowledge of the metaphysical heart that extends beyond its physical dimensions. There is a generous measure of wit, whimsy, attention to detail and instruction in her words. I feel this is her best book yet. It adds a seasoned and creative voice to the fields of medicine, nursing, clinical psychology and other caring professions. It is no passing book, but one that should be put on the top shelf and remain there."
~ David Morris, M.C., Board Certified Family Practice Physician and Credentialed HIV Specialist, American Academy of HIV Medicine

"Dr. Forrest has provided a much needed book for both caregivers and professionals in dealing with the many facets of dementias. She thoroughly and eloquently describes an array of illnesses that can result in cognitive decline. She has successfully blended practical information, research issues, and detailed descriptions of issues related to cognitive decline to help readers apply this knowledge. Additionally, she speaks to the very import issue of the spiritual aspects of dementing illnesses, an aspect that is too often overlooked. This book provides a wealth of information to anyone interest in learning more about the many faces of dementia and some of the current research questions that need to be pursued in the quest to unravel the ongoing mystery of cognitive impairment and decline."
~ Linda Blazina, Ph.D., Clinical Psychologist Private Practice, co-author of "The Psychopathology of Dementia" in *Handbook of Dementing Illnesses*, edited by John C. Morris, 1994.

TOUCH THE SPIRIT

Connecting to the Inner World of Dementia

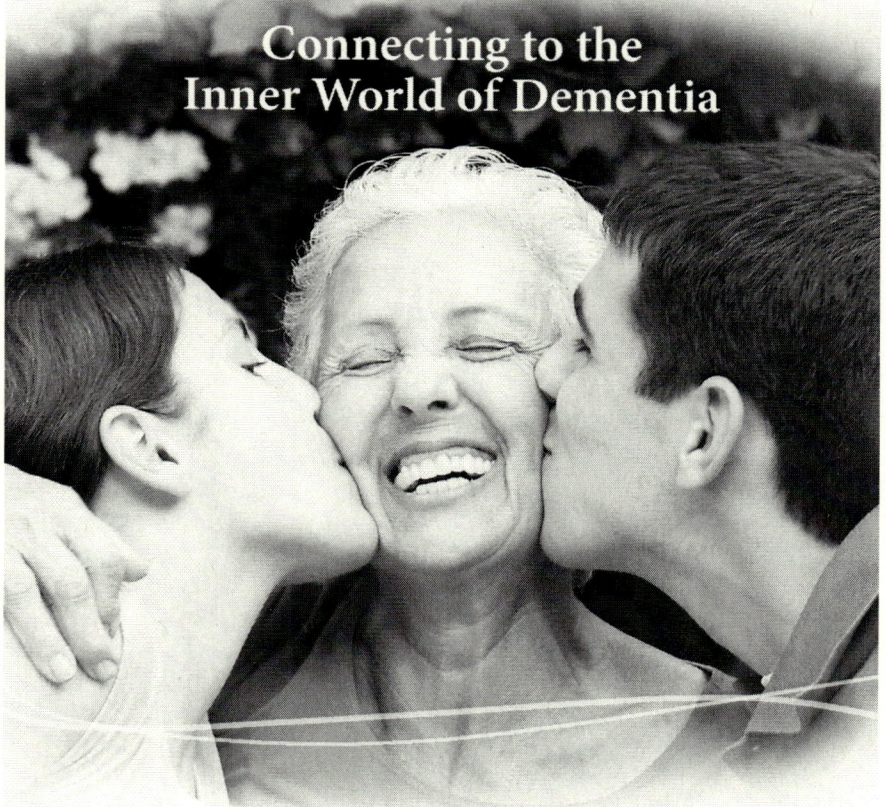

Deborah A. Forrest, Ph.D.
AUTHOR OF THE INTERNATIONAL BESTSELLER **SYMPHONY OF SPIRITS**

Butter Lamp Books • Greater Atlanta, Georgia

TOUCH THE SPIRIT: CONNECTING TO THE INNER WORLD OF DEMENTIA

Copyright © 2013 by Deborah A. Forrest. All rights reserved. Printed in the United States of America. No part of this book may be used or reproduced in any manner whatsoever without written permission except in the case of brief quotations embodied in critical articles or reviews. For information, address Butter Lamp Books, P.O. Box 2154, Jasper, Georgia 31043

www.butterlampbooks.com
Book Jacket designed by George Foster
Interior designed by Deborah Perdue, Illumination Graphics

Library of Congress Cataloging-in-Publication Data

Forrest, Deborah A.
Touch the Spirit: connecting to the world of dementia/ 1st ed.
ISBN-13   978-0-9860156-2-5
ISBN-10   0-9860156-2-8

Dementia – Alzheimer's disease – Multi-Infarct dementia –Stroke – Frontotemporal Lobe dementia – Lewy Body disease – Huntington's disease -AIDs – Parkinson's disease – Traumatic Brain Injuries – Shaken Brain Syndrome – Chronic Traumatic Encephalopathy -Age associated memory impairment – Chemobrain – Open heart surgery – Spirituality – Music – Art – Storytelling – Poetry – Humor – Sex - Prevention — Title

First Edition: June, 2013

OTHER BOOKS BY
DR. DEBORAH FORREST

*Symphony of Spirits:
Encounters with the Spiritual
Dimensions of Alzheimer's*

*Mela's Dream: A Story for Parents
Who Have Lost a Child*

~ DISCLAIMER ~

The material contained in this work is general in nature. The information is not provided as medical advice and should not be relied upon as such. If you need medical advice upon which you intend to rely, you should contact a physician. Neither the author of this work, nor the authors or providers of information contained in this document assume any responsibility for the actions or non-actions taken by those who have received information, and no one shall be entitled to a claim for detrimental reliance on any information provided or expressed.

Dr. Deborah A. Forrest

THIS BOOK IS DEDICATED TO

Kate Forrest Swaringen

The Eldest member of the Forrest Family of Western North Carolina
Born August 28, 1911
She continues to show us "how a vibrant spirit" can help one live for at least 100 years and beyond

And to the late

Robert J. Davis Sr.
(1923-2011)

My high school principal & American History teacher
During his later years, Mr. Davis always reminded me that my words can reach far beyond the pages of any book and touch people's lives in ways that I will never know

~ CONTENTS ~

Introduction xv

ONE: Our Connections Have Value 1

TWO: A Kaleidoscope of Dementias 11
    Normal Aging & Memory Loss 14
    Mild Cognitive Impairment 15
    Alzheimer's Disease 16
    Lewy Bodies Disease 18
    Vascular Dementia 19
    Parkinson's Disease 20
    Huntington's Disease 21
    Fronto-Temporal Lobe Dementia 22
    Traumatic Brain Injury Induced Dementia ... 25
    HIV/AIDS Dementia 29
    Chemotherapy Induced Dementia/Chemobrain 31
    Open Heart Surgery Induced Dementia 32

THREE: A Path to the Inner World of Dementia 37

FOUR: Soul Strings 51
    Music 51
    Painting & Drawing 56
    Reminiscence Therapy 57
    Storytelling 58
    Making Friends with the Enemy 59
    Heart-to-Heart Conversations 61
    Poetry 62
    Creative Cuing Environments 63
    Safe Havens 64

	Computers 66
	Animals, Aroma, & Children 66
	Humor 69
	Flash Cards 70
	Grieve the Losses & Celebrate the Assets 71
	Sex 74
FIVE:	**Threads of Dementia Prevention** 77
	Stress Management 83
	Swollen Ankles Management 83
	Foods 84
	Hormone Levels 85
	Sleep 85
	Social Circle 86
	Dental Care 86
	Vitamins 86
	Exercise 88
	Diabetes Prevention 88
	Vision & Hearing Care 90
	Memory Boosters 90
SIX:	**Caregivers: Our Unsung Heroes** 93
	Monetary Value of Caregiver Services 93
	Caregiver's Support 98
	Caregiver's Diet 100
	Caregiver's Sleep Options 101
	Caregiver's Stress Management 102
	TLC for Own Body 102
	Family Drama Issues 104
	Legal & Financial Documents 105
	Caregiver's Honoring of Self 106

INTRODUCTION

SEVEN: Dementia in the 21st Century 111
    Staggering Growth to Come 111
    Monetary Costs of Care 111
    New Research on Prevention & Treatments:
    Exercise 112
    Diet 113
    Hormone Therapies 115
    Gene Therapies 115

Epilogue 119

Acknowledgments 123

End Notes 124

Appendix 141

Recommended Reading 149

About the Author 153

Resources for Information on Dementias in the USA & Foreign Countries 155

"Believe"
Excerpt of lyrics by Ronnie Dunn & Craig Watson

I can't quote the book

The chapter or the verse

You can't tell me it all ends

In a slow ride in a hearse

You know I'm more and more convinced

The longer that I live

Yeah, this can't be

No, this can't be

No, this can't be

(Chorus)

When I raise my hands, bow my head

I'm finding more and more truth in the words written in red

They tell me that there's more to life than just what I can see

I believe

Oh, I

I believe

I believe

I believe

I believe

Permission granted by Sony Music

INTRODUCTION

The first time I heard Ronnie Dunn sing the song "I Believe," I got cold chills. Every time I hear it, I utter a silent "thank you" under my breath. That song so eloquently speaks to the presence of a human spirit—a soul! It causes the listener to stop and think for a moment about what happens to that soul when its time here is over. I agree with Ronnie Dunn. There is more to life than just what we see. Before "that slow ride in a hearse," there is a lot more the human spirit can accomplish than many people seem to realize. For me, this realization came in a rather traumatic way. Sometimes I don't "get it" when the Universe, God, the Creator, that Great Spirit in the sky tries to send me messages. When this happens, other steps are taken to make sure I stop and pay attention.

During the early 1990s, I was working as a staff nurse in an operating room and taking graduate courses for my PhD in clinical psychology during my off hours. Life was progressing smoothly. I was working at a steady job, taking graduate courses, and doubling up my career transition efforts with a weekend training course in cognitive therapy. My thoughts about the human spirit and people's souls were neatly tucked away in my memory banks. There they were confined to my memories of earlier years in my life when I had to cope with the death of my parents and many of the pediatric patients I cared for at the children's hospital where I worked as a young graduate nurse.

In the 1990s I was moving on to a new life and a new career. Graduate school IQ tests revealed that I had a "genius level" IQ. I was proud to learn that news. Not being the prettiest girl in my family or in any of my classes—anywhere—I was delighted to know that at least I had an exceptionally good brain working for me in this life. Little did I know that tiny bubble of joy was about to burst!

On a weekend trip home to Tennessee to attend my only niece's high school graduation, I was involved in a single-car accident. As my new shiny red compact car traveled down a long country road, my thoughts were focused on all of the schoolwork I had to do when I returned home. Suddenly, as my car topped a hill, I could see a line of cars ahead of me. All of them were stopped. "What do I do?" rushed through my head. The car immediately in front of me belonged to my baby sister. She was on her way to a business event nearby. In the passenger's seat was one of the managers from her restaurant. Quickly, I scanned the scene just in front of me. Off to my right, down a very steep ravine, was a huge grassy field with a group of children playing baseball. Off to my left was a steep grass-covered bank with a deep ditch in front of it. Without giving the situation any more thought, I hit the brakes and turned my little car toward the ditch. Surely it would just slide into the ditch and stop. I would be ok and no one would get hurt. My car would probably just come out with a few scratches and dent or two. That was what *I* thought! That is not what the Universe, God, the Creator, or the Great Leader of the Spirit World had in store for me.

As I mentioned earlier, it sometimes takes more than a little nudge to get me to pay attention to what I should be noticing. In this instance, it was going to take a lot. I was about to get a "smack up the side of the head" that would alter the world as I knew it!

Introduction

As my little car slid off the paved highway, it suddenly spun around. The tail end of the car was facing the line of traffic. At that point, I could see that my car was going to into the ditch and then hit an embankment on the passenger's side. Surely I would be OK was the last thought that I had.

Suddenly, from out of nowhere, I heard three voices speaking to me. "You are not going to die. Turn your head and shoulder into the door." There was no one else in the car but me! There was no time to think. I followed the instructions of those the unseen voices. As I leaned into the door, everything went black. I do not know how long I was unconscious. The near-death event that I experienced that day should have been enough to change my worldview. It does for most people. Not me! Apparently that guiding force knew I would need a stronger wake-up call. I had to undergo a closed-head injury and some contusions and cuts all over my body. That special IQ score I had cherished so much was altered forever. Life as I knew it was over.

Like so many of the soldiers returning from the wars of Iraq and Afghanistan, I was forced to deal with the damage that comes with a traumatically induced "Shaken Brain." In my case, all aspects of my speech, my comprehension skills, and my memory systems were permanently damaged. Although the neurologist who treated me weeks later told me the Post-Concussion Syndrome symptoms I was experiencing would clear up in about three months, only some of them did. Twenty years have passed since the motor-vehicle accident occurred. I have learned new and different ways to work with and adapt to the permanent cognitive changes I experienced that fateful day.

Like those war veterans with Shaken Brain Syndrome, I initially felt lost in the world. On the outside I looked normal. I had no major physical signs of trauma—only scratches from the shattered windshield. On the inside, nothing was ever going to be "normal" again. Nothing in my world made sense for the longest time. For months, my computer was my best friend. My speech was impaired for more than a year, and to cope with this problem, I began to communicate by typing. It was the early years of the Internet. I had friends across the country to interact with online. I could type simple sentences to people in the outside world. For a few moments out of each day, I felt normal again.

Over the weeks, months, and years that followed, my view of the world changed. Rather than relying on my old "photographic memory" to get me through life, I was forced to work with the strengths of my remaining brain tissue. For those areas that no longer worked well or at all, I had to come up with alternative strategies to get me through each day. Quickly, I learned that I could no longer use the "ten-dollar" words I had learned in college. Nor could I recite passages from books or research studies like I had once done as an accomplished scholar. I had to work with the language skills I had at that moment. This meant that I could speak using only simple words and simple phrases. This form of speech became the norm. Trying to remember anything beyond the here and now took practice. It never got easier. I finally gave up trying to remember most things. Today I carry notepads with me everywhere I go. I write down everything that I want to remember. The written word is my guide. This process remains ongoing. Coping with these changes has been frustrating—very frustrating some days. I still find myself constantly searching for new ways to trigger my memories and to repair the damages that were done. Some days I have to stop and remember that it is what it is, and that I must go on with life as it is now.

If I get a cold, a sinus infection, or the annual flu, my brain decompensates. This is "normal for me." Confusion sets in. My

Introduction

memory systems become seriously impaired. I am unable to work with numbers. My coping strategy is to withdraw until all systems return to "my new normal." Also, the damage to the left side of my brain left me with complete right-sided weakness from my head to my toes. So when I get overly stressed and extremely tired, my body speaks—not my brain. I drag the right side of my body anywhere I want to go. Again, my coping strategy is to withdraw and rest until I can regain my ability to carry myself upright and "unimpaired."

Sharing this private and very personal traumatic event with you is important. I want my readers to understand that I have an up-close and personal relationship with the condition known as dementia. Mine was created by a traumatic brain injury. This event makes me "at risk" for Alzheimer's disease. If that were not enough "risk" for one single life, I also have a strong family history of diabetes, strokes with vascular dementia, heart disease, and am now over the age of sixty years. My risk factors mount with each passing year. Rather than dwell on these, I continue to educate myself about the diseases of dementia. I keep up with literature about the new ways for preventing these diseases that come with age. I practice as many of them as I can. I try to listen to what my body tells me is "good and bad." And I consciously choose to look forward to living to be at least 102 years old. My dear cousin Kate has made it. I possess those genes. I am confident that I have many more years to enjoy life. Attitude and gratitude are two words I live by each day.

♪

In an effort to "make sense" of my tragedy, I began to learn about dementia and what it really is. As a part of my learning process, I began to work with Alzheimer's patients and their families. That experience led me to write my first book.

Nearly a dozen years have passed since that book, *Symphony of Spirits: Encounters with the Spiritual Dimensions of Alzheimer's*, was published. In it I shared my experiences of caring for seven remarkable patients suffering from Alzheimer's and other neurodegenerative diseases and the powerful process I underwent to learn how to interact with their spiritual dimensions. As I learned more about this aspect of each patient, I began to recognize a vital piece of life that still resided in each of them. My encounters with their spiritual dimensions gave me a new understanding of people with dementia and their illnesses. The wonderful women and men whose lives formed the basis for the experiences described in that book have passed on to the other side. Their families have moved on.

It is important for the families of the seven patients described in that book to know that their stories were read by people around the world. Their lives made an impact on others. The many letters and emails that I received from readers made it clear that their stories touched hearts. They helped to cast a new light on the world of Alzheimer's disease as well as the other disorders that can produce the condition known as dementia described in those stories.

The growth of Alzheimer's disease continues. As our global community ages, its prevalence is becoming even more noticeable to everyone—even those who would like to stick their heads in the sand and ignore it. Research into the cause(s) of Alzheimer's disease also continues. Some interesting theories about its origin have emerged from different research groups outside the United States. Still, no cure has been uncovered—yet. Fortunately, though, a new area of interest has emerged in the past few years—prevention. A variety of strategies for the prevention of illnesses like Alzheimer's are being explored by researchers around the world. All of this new information will be shared in the pages of this new book.

Beyond Alzheimer's disease, there are other medical disorders that can impair a person's cognitive faculties and create limitations on how he or she lives in society. These include but are not limited to strokes, traumatic head injuries, fronto-temporal-lobe dementia, Lewy body disease, AIDs dementia, Parkinson's disease, clinical depression, mild cognitive impairment (MCI) , chemobrain (a chemotherapy-induced dementia), post open-heart surgery dementia, and some forty or more lesser known disorders that can produce the condition known as dementia. It is the alteration and/or destruction of a person's mental faculties and loss of independence that seem to frighten so many—especially in the case of Alzheimer's disease.

While different research groups continue to search for the causes and cures of all conditions that can produce dementia beyond Alzheimer's, others are also turning their focus and research toward prevention efforts. Some of newer prevention strategies for these other conditions are also are also covered. Many of them are also still undergoing validation through research studies.

The same need to understand the different aspects of altered brain functioning that led me to the stories told in Symphony of Spirits: Encounters with the Spiritual Dimensions of Alzheimer's also led me to look at other people around the world who also have conditions that lead to dementia. This ongoing search led me to the creation of this book. Paramount among all who cope with this condition known as dementia is a *desire to remain connected to the people around them and to the outside world.* Equally important for their family members and caregivers is a *desire to create and maintain a connection with the person who resides in the inner world of dementia.*

Many of the people I met over the years have told me phenomenal stories of their loved ones. Their stories describe some of the threads that have held them together. Their stories have led me on a new journey to find new threads. The "new threads" I have discovered can be woven together with the "old threads" to create a new fabric of life for those who live within the world of dementia. This notion of *staying connected* to a person with dementia is important! It is important for everyone involved—whether the dementia is caused by Alzheimer's disease, by a stroke, by Parkinson's disease, by a traumatic brain injury, or by any of the plethora of other diseases in our society that can cause it.

A lovely woman with Lewy body dementia who lives in Germany coined the phrase "dementia-consciousness"[1] What does that phrase mean to you? How will it impact your everyday world? How will it impact our global society? How will it affect the growing numbers of older adults and young Iraq and Afghanistan war veterans coping with some form of a dementia process? How will these people operate in communities that do not understand this phenomenon? How can their strengths and weaknesses as valued human beings even be recognized? How do we begin to acknowledge the contributions they still have to make to their families, to their communities, to society as a whole?

Part of the answer to all of these questions involves education. We must help everyone at every level of our society understand what dementia is *and* what it is not. Within the pages that follow, I have attempted to help readers understand in clear and simple terms what dementia really is. I hope that readers will find at least one piece of information to help him or her understand that to stay connected to a

INTRODUCTION

person who is living with a dementia process. This may require some effort and exploration to find ways to make those connections. Look to the person's earlier life. Look at their passions. Look at those things that brought them joy. Reviving a connection to an old memory may be the simplest way. And the adventure to find new or different ways to connect may be the most fulfilling effort of all.

For some people, establishing connections may involve carrying on one-way conversations that will never be reciprocated. These are the most challenging connections. They can also be the most rewarding growth experiences, but one's expectations of such connections must be altered. These are some of the "silent gifts" of dementia. Receive them as such and be prepared to have your life enriched.

Deborah A. Forrest, Ph.D.,
M.S.N.

ONE

Our Connections Have Value

Oh my friend, it's not what they take away from you that counts, it's what you do with what you have left.

—Hubert Humphrey

"Dr. Forrest, will you please come back inside? The director wants to speak to you for a moment." The voice belonged to the secretary for the local Alzheimer's Association, where I had just completed a presentation. She was standing in the doorway at the back of the building.

"Sure," I replied.

At that moment, I was ready to leave that Alzheimer's Association chapter's office and head toward my next speaking engagement. "What could he possibly want with me?" I thought to myself. "My presentation is over. I picked up the last of my papers and handouts. My bags and slides are right here in the trunk of my rental car. Oh well, I will see what he wants and then I can get on my way."

As I entered the director's office, I could see his face was beaming. I was puzzled. It must have shown on my face.

"Dr. Forrest, do you remember the man in the back of the room with the wavy white hair who kept asking you questions at the end of your presentation?"

"Yes," I replied.

"He came into my office after you left and gave us a check for one million dollars!" The director squealed with joy. The smile on his face lit up the room.

"What?" I could not understand what was happening. "Why?"

"He gave us this check for one million dollars because he liked your presentation!" the young man replied. "When he handed me the check, he told me that he wanted to support an Alzheimer's chapter that was willing to bring in speakers like you! He appreciated your honesty, your openness, your enthusiasm, and most of all your willingness to acknowledge that you did not have all of the answers. He also told me that he liked your presentation on spirituality. It was not restricted to any one line of religious thought or spiritual ideology. Your information allowed everyone in the room to take the ideas presented and use them within their own belief system. He really liked that. It gave him a comfort that he had not experienced up to that point. His wife has Alzheimer's. He has been taking care of her at home for quite a number of years."

As the Director continued to talk about how grateful they were for my presentation and for the donation they had just received, I was still reeling. Shock had overtaken my brain. It was hard for me to wrap my head around the idea that someone would give these people *one million dollars* because of what I said.

After several minutes of watching his mouth move, I could finally hear the rest of the story he was telling. This particular chapter's staff had tried on several different occasions to get this same man to make

ONE: OUR CONNECTIONS HAVE VALUES

a *simple small donation* to their group with no success. Like me, they were in complete shock when this extremely wealthy man came forth, unexpectedly, to make this very large contribution.

The gifting of a check for one million dollars was not the only surprise I encountered when *Symphony of Spirits: Encounters with the Spiritual Dimensions of Alzheimer's* first came out. During the early days of my cross-country travels to promote my book, I made a rare unscheduled stop over at my home in Georgia. On that very day, the telephone rang. The voice on the other end of the line was warm and friendly, and I recognized it immediately. Mr. Davis, my high school principal was calling to talk. Soon after the book was published, I had sent him a personal copy for his library. He had always been a big supporter of my accomplishments over the years, long after I had graduated and moved away. I wanted to share this important event with him.

"Hello, Debbie. This is Bob Davis. I just finished reading your book! I just had to call you and tell you how much I enjoyed reading it." There was an excitement in his voice that I had never heard. I could hardly get in a simple "Hello, Mr. Davis" before he was talking again.

"I have to go to nursing homes a lot to visit people I have known over the years—all types of people. I never knew what to say to them, especially the ones with Alzheimer's. NOW I KNOW what to do!" he said. The excitement in his voice was palpable. "After reading your book, I can be more comfortable visiting those people at the nursing homes. I can talk to their spirits! Thank you for sharing that with me."

His voice and his words stuck in my heart and in my mind. I was proud to be able to "give something back" to a man who had done so much for me in my life. Not too long after that telephone conversation, Mr. Davis and his dear wife, Lula, attended a book-signing event held for me in my hometown. Little did I know then that it would be the last time I would see them together. After that encounter, I would talk to Mr. Davis by telephone from time to time. On one of those phone calls, he mentioned that my book's content had occasioned some rather stimulating conversations between his grown children and his wife and him.

Life happened and we did not for talk for several years. In 2010 a mutual friend contacted me to inform me that Lula had passed away. I was devastated. She and Bob were like family to me. At the funeral I learned that she had been in a nursing home for two years and had died of some form of dementia—they thought it was Alzheimer's. I was shocked by this news. In all of my life, I never anticipated that Alzheimer's would touch the lives of either Bob or Lula Davis. Like so many, I thought, "It's supposed to happen to other people—not my friends." Bob Davis was never supposed to have a personal reason to use any of my information on Alzheimer's—especially for Lula, the love of his life. The value of what I had shared with him years earlier would take on a new meaning after Lula's funeral.

A couple of weeks after Lula's funeral, I picked up the telephone and called Bob Davis. He had been so grief stricken during the funeral I did not have an opportunity to talk with him. I did not want to let any more time pass between us.

"Hi Bob. It's Debbie Forrest," I said. "I don't know if you remember, but I spoke to you at the cemetery. You looked pretty worn out. I am so sorry that Lula has passed on."

"You did? Oh. Thank you." Bob replied. "That was a pretty rough time. Did I speak to you?"

"Yes, you did."

Like every telephone conversation before, Bob continued to talk without much interruption by me. "Good. Yes, Lula was sick for two years. I drove to the nursing home every day of those two years—except for two days when I had a cold. We talked every day. What is your telephone number? I tried to call you during those years but I could not find your number."

"Bob, I am so sorry we lost touch. I have moved to the mountains of North Georgia," I said. "Here is my new telephone number."

"What is that number again? Let me get my caregiver. I don't remember words and numbers very well anymore." Bob turned to his in-home caregiver to help him write down my new telephone number. "Now, I have that written down. We will have to stay in touch." Bob's vocabulary was interrupted by lapses for the word he was searching for. His memory was keen for some things—like the time he had spent with Lula. The stress of his recent loss was clearly taking a toll on his ability to discuss other topics we usually covered in our conversations. We ended the conversation with plans for future telephone conversations.

There was one more telephone conversation that followed that one. We talked about plans to spend time some together during the Christmas holidays of 2010. A heavy snowstorm prevented that meeting. He was in Nashville with his son and their family, and I was snowed in for days in Gatlinburg with my sister Becky and her new dog. I kept telling myself, "I will call Mr. Davis after the first of the new year when the snows melt, and we are both at home."

Months passed. I never got around to making that telephone call to Mr. Davis in the new year. Less than one year after Lula's passing, my dear friend contacted me again with more news. Bob Davis had joined his wife. This time I was devastated. My time with Mr. Davis had run out. Now two very important people who had been part of my life for more than fifty years were gone. It did not matter that I only saw them from time to time. They were part of the "fabric of my life." They had outlived my own parents, all of my aunts and uncles, and even my own husband. They had always been there for me. The value of their friendship, love, and support and the times we shared is incalculable! The fact that their lives were touched by dementia has left me with an indescribable sense of emptiness, though I am forever grateful that I was blessed to have them in my life.

Over the years people contacted to me to share their own stories of life with Alzheimer's. They were eager to describe some of benefits they derived from reading about the spiritual dimensions of Alzheimer's. Their stories were touched by threads of joy. Many thanked me for putting a voice to the spiritual aspect of dementia. Time and again they would say, "I don't feel crazy any more. Thank you." Here are some of the most memorable responses I received.

> *Just finished reading your book, AND I LOVED IT! I have been looking for just such an item. I have been working with Alzheimer's and people with Dementia for about 12 years. I have also worked with people with T.B.I. and M.R. as well as others with Dual Diagnoses....I have found spirituality to be a common denominator in many people as a treatment option.*
> Rev. Dr. T. S., Florida

> *My mother died from complications of AD in 1996...your book has given me a different and special take on the elderly who have dementia and I really appreciate that. It is one of the most difficult and painful things in life to watch a person lose everything so dear to them with this disease.*
> D. C., Utah

ONE: OUR CONNECTIONS HAVE VALUES

> *My 90 year old mother suffered a stroke that left her unable to speak. My sister and I have tried to honor her wishes for care during her 12 years in an area nursing home....I just wanted to let you know that after corresponding with you, I talked to my sister again and also gave her the book* Symphony of Spirits *to read. I also spoke to Mom Sunday with more ease than I have in a long time. She is and always has been a strong willed determined woman. This spirit has not forsaken her, and, perhaps, has gotten even stronger as she has had to fight so many physical problems. I told her that I loved her for her spirit and knew that she was still in there fighting, but if she is getting tired, it was ok to let go...both Ann [my sister] and I would understand. It was one of the most honest discussions I have had with Mom. I did not see any signs that she understood, but I felt better after the situation.*
>
> K. P.

W.B., the wonderful daughter of a mother with Alzheimer's, sent me the most beautiful story about her mother and the times they shared during the ten years she took care of her. She made clear to me the value of addressing the spiritual dimension in persons with dementia:

> *When I heard you speak in May [at an Alzheimer's Conference], I knew I was not alone in my connection with spirits and Alzheimer's. Thank you for coming forth and sharing your stories. It is so very helpful to the rest of us who, in the face of others, appear to have lost it....I read your book like it was a textbook. I underlined, commented, contemplated and reread passages to firmly implant the ideas and connect it with ideas I already had. I do not remember*

reading with such energy. I think it took an hour and a half to read the first 26 pages…you certainly had me hooked."

As she shared more pieces of her time with her mother, I was beyond thrilled when I read the following:

….it hit me, lucky for me (and I am serious about the luck) I "got" Mom the last 10 years of her life. I was able to be with her from the day I suspected the disease to the last. What a gift I received.
W. B., Oregon

When individuals read about the spiritual dimension of Alzheimer's many would respond like this caregiver from Canada. In each instance there was a personal sense of validation about the spiritual dimension of life.

I just read your book. I couldn't put it down once I started. My father was recently diagnosed with Alzheimer's. He is 77 years old [in 2004] and has had some symptoms of dementia for the past 6 years. He is just past the early stages with some problems with language, abstract thinking, poor judgment and changes in behavior. I read your book hoping for further understanding of how to be there for him and my mother. I was pleased to learn about spirituality. Thank you for your book. It's nice to know that spirituality is a part of me (I'm not going crazy) as it is for everyone.
P. B., Canada

Marilyn S., a friend of mine who is a nurse at a large hospital in California, told me that reading *Symphony of Spirits* "changed the way" she now thinks about patients with dementia. She shared with me a portion of an experience one of her colleagues there in the hospital recounted to her:

> ...*today I even encouraged a nursing assistant to talk to the (Alzheimer's) patient's spirit after she told me about the patient's "look in her eyes"—that she was trying to tell her something. I asked her what she thought the patient was trying to say. Without missing a beat, she said, "Let me go. I want to leave this world and cross over to the other side, but my son won't let me go. He is afraid to live his life without me. He keeps holding on to me."*

R. M., a Native American elder I met in a bookstore during my travels, spent one afternoon talking to me at length about some of the lessons of the "Spirit World" his tribal elders had taught. Sometime after that meeting, he wrote to me. His message contained some very important words that will make more sense in later chapters. He wrote, "The Creator gave us two ears and one mouth, so we could hear twice as much as we speak. You and your book (*Symphony of Spirits*) show this to be a common theme, and bring smiles to my face, as this is how we learn. Remember too, the heart has ears. It can hear. It will carry messages to the head."

This simple meeting with one wise Native American elder changed *my life*. It provided me with a powerful message that made sense—on a gut level. It was that "missing link" I was seeking. His message gave me an image that I understood. The heart is a powerful organ. It could be "a doorway" to the human soul. For years I read books about people's responses to a heart filled with love, to a heart's code, to a broken heart, and to a healing heart. Maybe there was really something to this idea that a "heart can hear ." Ten more years would pass before

I learned about the neurological underpinnings of this message. The heart and head have a major nerve that carries messages from the heart to the head and back. This "neuro-cardiology connection" – as my friend Dr. David Morris calls it – involves a very sophisticated feedback loop, the sympathetic nervous system, adrenal catecholamines, beta receptors, calcium channels as well as other intricate processes. Even though I had studied this neural connection in several anatomy classes during my different years in school, I did not grasp the importance of this single nerve. It took a series of research presentations about the biological basis of compassion for me to grasp one single concept. In their efforts to demonstrate compassion within the human body, the researchers described a communication pathway between the heart and the brain that is related to compassion. In an instant I had an "aha moment." The "heart really can hear." When the heart is stimulated, it carries a nerve impulse to the brain. The brain processes that impulse. For the purposes of this book, I will stop here and simply acknowledge that there is biological process that is associated with heart communications. These stories from family members and friends demonstrate the value of making connections with others—in this case, with persons who have Alzheimer's. They are varied in content as well as meaning, and they will have value for some but not for others.

The value of learning about spirituality and its integral relationship to the world of dementia will be different for everyone. Some will find it useful. Others will not. No two people will have the same experience regardless of the situation. The value of recognizing there is a doorway into the heart and soul of the person with dementia is a personal one. The decision to utilize that doorway is also an individual choice. For people who have been compromised by diseases of aging such as Alzheimer's, strokes, traumatic brain injuries (TBI), or Pick's disease, the resulting connections can be powerful and rewarding.

TWO

A Kaleidoscope of Dementias

Who is your enemy? Mind is your enemy.
Who is your friend? Mind is your friend.
Learn the ways of the mind. Tend the mind with care.

—Buddha

Dementia is a growing phenomenon. It can occur at any time in one's life. It is not just a condition of aging. Not everyone will develop it with age. It does not discriminate—against anyone, anywhere. It knows no boundaries. Its causes are as diverse as the kaleidoscope of symptoms it can present. Over the coming decades, dementia will become one of the greatest social equalizers on earth.

The very word *dementia* strikes fear in the hearts of men and women everywhere. For some like me who are willing to let "that word" flow from our mouths, the risk of rejection parallels that of someone with leprosy. Why? Many still hold an archaic belief they can "catch it!" They will go out of their way to avoid anyone or anything that "might cause them to catch dementia." After all, it is linked to other fearful concepts like being feeble, mindless, old, and senile, and to dying. And for many, dementia is *only* associated with the dreaded Alzheimer's disease.

This is our reality in the twenty-first century! Why? Very few people in the world know the meaning of the word dementia. Even fewer understand what it is and is not.

Virtually only a handful of people—in the grand scheme of things—seem to know dementia can be created by a variety of different medical conditions, not just Alzheimer's. In an effort to educate readers about dementia and what disorders can produce it, a brief review of the most common disorders and/or conditions will follow. More detailed information can be obtained from the organizations listed in the Resources section at the end of this book. Over the years many well-meaning friends and colleagues have said to me, "Deborah, stop giving us all of this technical information. People can read about that stuff in books. Just tell us your stories. We love your stories." While this may be true for many, I am aware that many people in this country and in others around the world do not have easy access to books or to the internet. Getting even the most basic medical and technical information about any of the diseases or conditions that can produce dementia can be a challenge. For some it is impossible. In this global society where social media is changing our communication styles and access to knowledge, I am very much aware that there are still many people in near and far-away places living without computers, smart phones, libraries, or any of the other information outlets the rest of us now take for granted.

Still, they have loved ones who succumb to the disorders that can produce dementia. This chapter is for those people. It contains basic information that is written in a simple and concrete format. Why? People with dementia cannot comprehend or understand complex

Two: A Kaleidoscope of Dementias

sentences and abstract concepts. People working with them must develop communicate styles that use simple, words which are clear and concrete. This approach will allow everyone to operate on the same playing field. Communication will become clearer for everyone!

This brief overview must begin with a basic description of dementia. *Dementia is a generic term for a constellation of symptoms that are associated with a variety of disorders*[2]. It is frequently associated with several age-related illnesses like Alzheimer's, Lewy body disease, vascular dementia (strokes), Huntington's disease, Parkinson's disease, fronto-templar dementia, or Pick's diseases. It can also be created by a variety of traumatically induced brain injuries—for example, "shaken brain syndrome," sports injuries, multiple blows to the head, and motor vehicle accidents of any type. In short, for the latter category, any event that produces repeated blows to the head or a shaking of the brain inside the skull can over time produce a form of dementia.

Evidence is slowing emerging within the medical community that indicates patients who are undergoing some types of chemotherapy treatments and certain forms of open heart surgery are presenting with significant cognitive and behavioral changes.[3, 4] Many within these two newer groups of patients are dealing with a medically induced form of dementia. Because each human brain is as unique as that person's fingerprints, the presentation of dementia will vary from person to person as much as it will vary by the condition that created it.

For a more detailed description of dementia, we can go to a common medical dictionary used by physicians. In it defines dementia as "an organic mental syndrome characterized by a general loss of intellectual abilities involving impairment of memory, judgment, and abstract thinking as well as changes in personality. It does not include loss of intellectual functioning caused by a clouding of consciousness (as in delirium – an acute reversible organic mental syndrome) nor that caused by depression or other functional mental disorder (pseudodementia). Dementia may be caused by a large number of conditions, some reversible and some progressive, that cause widespread cerebral damage or dysfunction. The most common cause of dementia is Alzheimer's disease[5].

NORMAL AGING AND MEMORY LOSS

"I can't remember things like I used to. Oh My God, am I getting Alzheimer's?" This is a common question I hear from people over fifty years of age. When I tell them it is probably a normal part of their aging process or the result of some stressful event they have been dealing with, a look of relief quickly sweeps across their faces.

Listen, folks, some memory loss *is* a part of the normal aging process. The decline most people can expect in this part of life typically affects their long-term memory or recent memory (*secondary memory*) more so than it does their short-term (*immediate*) memory or remote (*tertiary*) memory[6]. In other words, you are more likely to remember events from a long time ago over things that just happened a few seconds or a few minutes ago. Retrieving any of the information in your memory systems will take longer to access. These are affectionately known as "senior moments ." These "senior moments" do pass and the information sought does surface—eventually. Keep in mind that although the processes involved in our brain's capacity for remembering become less effective as we grow older, the content of our memories (our base of knowledge) can and does continue to increase. Now breathe!

MILD COGNITIVE IMPAIRMENT

Mild cognitive impairment (MCI) is a relatively new term in the field of aging[7]. It used to be called age associated memory impairment or AAMI. The term MCI was created by medical experts to designate an intermediate stage between the cognitive decline of normal aging and the more pronounced decline of dementia. It is an "in between stage of memory loss" that the experts are exploring. It doesn't always lead to Alzheimer's disease, and they are continuing to look into this area.[8,9] Recent media interviews with international singing legend Glen Campbell and his wife, for example, suggest that Mr. Campbell was showing signs of MCI before he was ultimately diagnosed with Alzheimer's disease. It is interesting to see Mr. Campbell on his world tour and performing with his family—after being diagnosed with Alzheimer's disease. This is an excellent public example of how one family is working with the *strengths* of this man who has Alzheimer's disease and *adapting to the weaknesses* created by his memory loss.

On the surface of MCI, the person will experience problems with memory, language, thinking, and judgment that are greater than those typically seen with normal age-related changes. A person and his/her family and friends may be aware that the individual's memory and/or other mental functions have changed. Generally, though, the changes noticed are not severe enough to interfere with the person's daily life and usual activities.

Experts at the Mayo Clinic point out that the presence of mild cognitive impairment increases a person's risk of developing dementia – including Alzheimer's – if the main problem is with memory. They also want people to know that some people with mild cognitive impairment *never* get worse and some eventually do get better.[10]

DEMENTIA OF THE ALZHEIMER'S TYPE

This was the phrasing used by Pat Head Summitt, Head Coach of the University of Tennessee Woman's Basketball Coach, during the summer of 2011, when she announced to the world that she had received a diagnosis of "early onset Alzheimer's disease" by the doctors at the Mayo Clinic.[11] Only a few weeks later, Glen Campbell announced that he too had received a diagnosis of Alzheimer's disease.[12] Both made it clear to the world that their lives would continue. Pat Summitt continued to coach her stellar team of accomplished women with the help of a group of loyal staff who had worked with her for many years. They helped her *adapt to the weaknesses* the Alzheimer's had created and *supported her many strengths* that allowed her to continue with her coaching duties as the most successful basketball coach in history. At the conclusion of her 2011-2012 season, she made the decision to step down from her job at the university and focus her attentions on the Pat Head Summit Alzheimer's Disease Foundation. As mentioned earlier, in 2011 Glen Campbell and his wife and children engaged in a worldwide tour to promote his final and most well received CD ever—despite a diagnosis of Alzheimer's. With the tour completed, Glen Campbell continues to perform his music in smaller venues. Life goes on.

These families and friends of the famous and not famous work each day with a multitude of cognitive and behavior changes that come over time with this disease. There are good days and there are rough days for everyone. Alzheimer's disease clearly does not discriminate. But because this particular disease moves across the human brain in a very individualized manner, no two people will experience exactly the same changes at the same time; nor will each person display the same symptoms in any uniform pattern. Even the disease's rate of progression will vary—from two years to twenty years!

What does dementia of the Alzheimer's type look like on the surface?

We have been told for decades that it unfolds in three stages: early, middle, and final. The common trends include memory problems that get worse over time, with a progression to an inability to care for oneself and an inability to recognize familiar people and places. Finally, death comes to put an end to this dreadful disease.

Over the past decade, researchers have gained a better understanding of the progression of Alzheimer's. Dr. Barry Reisenberg and his colleagues at the New York University School of Medicine's Silberstein Aging and Dementia Research Center now believe there are "Seven Stages of Alzheimer's."[13] They have created a new framework of understanding for doctors and caregivers to use. It will allow everyone to be able work from a common set of guidelines. These guidelines are designed to show how a person's abilities will change from normal functioning through the advanced stages of Alzheimer's. For a short review of the new Seven Stages of Alzheimer's, see the Resources section at the end of this book. Take time to look over this information. It is important that everyone is working with this same foundational level of information.

Even though we now have these guidelines for the Seven Stages of Alzheimer's available to us, there are still events not covered in these new guidelines that can serve as *red flags* to alert loved ones to the possibility of an Alzheimer's diagnosis. One common problem occurs when the person starts to complain of having difficulty following the conversations of others. Another problem is poor judgment with finances. The person may buy things they don't need or noticeably give away large sums of money to telemarketers, religious groups, or con men who come to their doors. A major problem can be mood changes that were not previously seen in the person. Confusion, suspiciousness, fear, or unusual signs of anxiety can be markers that something is wrong. Finally, if the person complains about poor memory that is getting worse from year to year, an evaluation by a neurologist is probably warranted.

On a positive note, thanks to the early diagnosis of Alzheimer's disease and the growing variety of allopathic and alternative treatments that are now available, many people are living high-quality lives for many years before any major decline in function necessitates alterations to their daily activities.

DEMENTIA WITH LEWY BODIES

Lewy body dementia (LBD) is not a rare disease: It affects nearly 1.3 million Americans. Its prevalence in other parts of the world is unknown at this point. Symptoms of Lewy body disease closely resemble those of Alzheimer's disease and Parkinson's disease. Often it is difficult for the doctor to make a definitive diagnosis of Lewy body disease because the symptoms of these three diseases are so similar. According to the Lewy Body Dementia Association, DLB or "dementia with Lewy bodies" is caused by a build-up of Lewy bodies -accumulated bits of alpha-synuclein protein-in an area of the brain that controls particular aspects of memory and motor control. Its symptoms include a progressive cognitive decline combined with three defining features: (1) pronounced fluctuations in alertness and attention such as frequent drowsiness, periods of time spent staring into space or disorganized speech, (2) recurrent visual hallucinations, and (3) Parkinsonian motor symptoms such as rigidity and the loss of spontaneous movement.[14] While there is no cure for dementia with Lewy bodies, early diagnosis and a comprehensive medical treatment approach can extend the quality of life and independence for individuals with this diagnosis.

VASCULAR DEMENTIA

Vascular dementia is the second most common type of dementia – after Alzheimer's disease.[15] This condition can occur after a single major stroke blocks a large blood vessel and cuts off the blood supply to a significant part of the brain that it feeds. In this situation, the condition is referred to as "post-stroke dementia." The other vascular event that can produce a vascular dementia occurs when a series of small strokes or infarcts block small blood vessels in the brain. While these small strokes do not cause major symptoms in and among themselves, over time their cumulative or combined effects become noticeable. This condition is known as multi-infarct dementia.[16]

The symptoms of a vascular dementia can and will vary depending upon the specific areas of the brain that are deprived of blood. The impairments may occur in "steps," where there is a fairly sudden and noticeable change in functioning rather than the slow decline seen in Alzheimer's. Medical professionals sometimes refer to these changes as a "stepwise" progression of alterations in functioning that are "patchy" in appearance.[17]

Persons who are vulnerable to a vascular dementia may have had a heart attack. Others, like me, have high blood pressure, high cholesterol, hardening of the arteries, and/or may be at risk for diabetes. Still other hereditary risk factors for heart disease are often present.[18]

The clinical presentation of vascular dementia will look different for each person, in part due to the location and type of the stroke as well as the number of strokes experienced. The symptoms seen with this type of dementia can include:

- Confusion, which may get worse at night
- Memory problems; these may or may not be present depending upon whether or not the brain regions important for memory are affected

- Difficulties with concentration, planning, communicating, and following instructions or commands
- Reduced or lowered ability to carry out daily activities
- Physical symptoms frequently seen during the early phase of a stroke include sudden weakness in one or more limbs, difficulty speaking, and/or confusion[19]

Individuals who experience a vascular event that leads to a dementia process can still live vibrant and productive lives, as evidenced by such people as the award winning movie legend Kirk Douglas, who suffered a major stroke several years ago. Mr. Douglas remains active within the film industry and is often seen making public appearances with his wife and other members of his family.

PARKINSON'S DISEASE

Michael J. Fox, another award-winning actor, has become the face of Parkinson's disease in America. His willingness to withhold his own medications—prior to his testimony before the US Congress in order to show Congress and the world his tremors—is both brave and admirable. His continued efforts to secure funding to find a cure for Parkinson's have raised the public visibility of this disease. Even now, he is holding public Internet forums to educate people about Parkinson's disease and to recruit people for ongoing research studies.[20]

While Parkinson's disease is known for its symptoms involving movement, coordination, physical task challenges, and mobility issues, most people are unaware of the "non-motor symptoms" that may be more troublesome than the motor impairments. These include sleep disturbances, fatigue, and loss of energy, depression, fear and anxieties, vision and dental problems, sexual problems, and impulsive behaviors that are brought on as side effects of the medications that people with the disease must take.[21]

In some cases, persons with Parkinson's disease may also experience dementia. The cognitive issues facing this group of people include memory difficulties, slowed thinking processes, and confusion.[22] For more detailed information on what is happening with Parkinson's disease research, please consult the Resources section at the end of this book.

HUNTINGTON'S DISEASE

Like Parkinson's, Huntington's disease—a genetically transmitted disorder—is known for its progressive decline in motor functioning. Like Alzheimer's disease, the decline associated with Huntington's is usually divided into stages.[23] In the first stage, there are subtle changes in coordination and involuntary movements. Depression and an irritable mood are frequently present. The first signs of cognitive difficulties may appear in the form of difficulty thinking through problems.

In the middle stage, the movement disorder may become more of a problem. Activities of daily living require assistance. Diminished speech and swallowing difficulties only add to the person's daily challenges. In this stage, the person will experience a further decline in cognitive functioning as the abilities to think and reason clearly become impaired.

In the final stage, the person with Huntington's becomes totally dependent on others for everything. The abilities to walk and talk are gone. Although the person's cognitive functioning is significantly impaired to qualify as having some form of dementia, the ability to comprehend language and recognize family and friends is retained. Sadly, there is no cure for this disease. For information on support services for patients with this disease and their caregivers, please see the Resources section of this book.

FRONTO-TEMPORAL DEMENTIA

Fronto-temporal dementia (FTD) is a new term within the medical community. It is an umbrella term that is used to describe a large number of clinical syndromes that are associated with the shrinking of the frontal and temporal anterior lobes of the brain.[24] Experts in this area designate Pick's disease, primary progressive aphasia, and semantic dementia as members of this clinical syndrome. Others are proposing to add cortico-basal degeneration and progressive supranuclear palsy to this syndrome. It is important for readers to know that the distinctions among these syndromes are hazy and an accurate diagnosis can only be made after death.

While fronto-temporal dementias were initially thought to be rare, experts now believe they are equally as common as Alzheimer's in persons under the age of sixty-five.[25] Given this newest information, the devastation these progressively degenerating diseases bring to patients and their families is worthy of some added attention in this chapter.

The diseases that create FTL dementia attack the parts of the brain that are responsible for judgment, empathy, and social behavior. Individuals stricken with FTD often develop personality changes, make disastrous financial decisions, become sexually inappropriate, and/or engage in compulsive behaviors. In some forms of FTD, the person's speech is lost, while others produce impairment in movements similar to Parkinson's disease and amyotrophic lateral sclerosis (ALS) or Lou Gehrig's disease.[26]

The onset of any of the diseases of FTD is usually between the ages of forty and sixty years of age. While there are fewer problems with memory, the behavioral changes can be devastating to the families of the patient as well as to co-workers. Because the patient looks normal, those around the individual often do not realize there is a problem. Family members, especially the spouse, become isolated as friends, co-workers, and extended family members withdraw from contact with the afflicted person because he or she begins to display personality changes, make sexually inappropriate comments, engage in compulsive behaviors, become rude to others, and seem indifferent to what would seem to be mortifying to a healthy person.[27]

A description of Pick's disease, one of the more prominent syndromes of the FTD family, is offered here by a General Medical Practitioner who has been living with it for about ten years. This story will probably give readers a better understanding of what FTD truly does to a family. The following is a "brief run-down" of the features of Pick's disease according to his experience:[28]

> *The onset, unlike Alzheimer's disease, is usually between 50 and 60. Men and women are said to be affected equally, though you wouldn't think so if you have anything to do with the support group. Here the carers all seem to be the wives of suffers, with very few husbands seeking support. We think this just reflects the different way men go about seeking help, or rather, not seeking help. There is a family history quite commonly, though not in my case.*
>
> *It is a disease which affects the personality and social behavior. Memory is affected but it's not the salient feature that it is in Alzheimer's disease. So, considering the personality changes the sufferer may become more outgoing, or conversely—withdrawn. He may lose the ability to empathize with others, becoming a cold fish, and being selfish and unfeeling. Aggressive behavior may*

develop. He becomes less flexible, and will be irritated by being contradicted. He may develop obsessive routines, or get over absorbed in one particular idea—what in my case I call "getting a bee in my bonnet." He may lose his inhibitions and become sexually inappropriate. In other ways he may become inappropriate, making tactless comments, joking at the wrong moment or being rude, and generally being an anxiety and embarrassment to his wife.

Failure at work is often an early symptom, and is caused by the loss of the ability to make good decisions; also by the inability to notice changing circumstances, or if he has actually noticed something has changed—he fails to act on it. So the businessman notices his junior is spending the company's money wildly, but does nothing. The doctor notices a lump but takes no action.

Failure at work is also caused by loss of concentration, or by loss of social skills. I can't see when I am irritating someone. Another disastrous feature is that the sufferer may become a spendthrift. And finally, memory lapses will inevitably affect one's work performance. An important feature of the disease is loss of driving skills. This seems to be brought about by a mixture of loss of judgment together with an inability to be aware of peripheral things when the attention is focused to the front. Speech problems are a feature, and in true Pick's disease the sufferer ends up mute. An odd feature sometimes seen is overeating—simply stuffing one's face, and boozing. Other oddities are being unable to see things under one's nose; giving an opposite answer to that intended. [I am asked] "coffee or tea?" and I say "tea" when I mean "coffee." Lack of drive is common. Needing more sleep and falling asleep frequently

> *during the day may be a feature. Increased sensitivity to pain or temperature may also occur. My family complain that I have a "Pick's face"[:] I frequently have a cold, hard look, when I am anxious, agitated, or am just in a thoroughly bad mood, but sometimes this face in no way reflects how I am feeling at all. I occasionally catch this face in the mirror and I can see why it upsets the family because it just isn't me at all.* [28]

This eloquent doctor goes on to stress that many people expect his Pick's disease to look something like Alzheimer's disease, when in fact it does not. In the early stage of Pick's disease or any of the FTDs, the symptoms are nothing like those found in Alzheimer's. In this man's case, his extraordinary detachment from his condition allows him to talk about it as if it were happening to someone else. For some this presentation can be unnerving. To others, he appears to be a fraud trying to escape some bad deed. Regardless of anyone's opinion, this man is living with this disease, and he wants to others to know what it looks like from his medically trained perspective.

TRAUMATIC BRAIN INJURY INDUCED DEMENTIA

There are a vast number of ways one can sustain a traumatic brain injury: motor vehicle accidents, football injuries, boxing, soccer, improvised explosive device (IED) explosions, a single blow to the head from any object, a rapid shaking of the head and neck—just to name a few. As with the other conditions discussed in this chapter, the area of the brain impacted by the trauma will create the cognitive problems that follow. If the traumatic injury causes the brain to shake inside the skull, the injuries will involve both the site of impact as well as structures on the opposite side; this condition is referred to as "contra cue" damage. The person can experience a host of cognitive changes that result from multiple areas of the brain being shaken about inside the skull. In many cases, if the trauma is minimal, the person may suffer from a condition known as "post-concussion syndrome," which lasts for approximately three months. Persons with post-concussion syndrome will usually return to some level of their pre-injury functioning.[29]

It is important to note here that medical researchers have learned that each hit to the head causes a stretching of axons in the brain, even in concussions. When axons—the brain's communication system—are stretched, their inner lining is damaged.[30] Additionally, a variety of neurochemical changes also occur in the brain. These changes can produce disturbing behaviors that include such things as unprovoked fear responses, anxiety attacks, depression, short- and long-term memory problems, and increased irritability. Many will experience problems with sleep, and tiring out more easily is common. Over time these problem areas will subside as the brain heals. Some will disappear completely while others, such as tiring easily, will remain. Unfortunately, with each blow to the head that follows, more stretched axons and damage to the inner linings to the person's brain builds up. There is a cumulative effect with each blow to the head. Eventually the person will begin to show signs of cognitive problems. These problems can and will contribute to the onset of different presentations of dementia.[31,32,33]

A vocal group of retired professional football players with debilitating dementias are now demanding answers from their former major league football owners. They contend that the repeated hits to their heads during weekly games caused repeated traumatic brain injuries. Those traumatic brain injuries led to the debilitating dementias they are now forced to live with. Using their notoriety, this group of famous athletes is bringing the problem of repeated traumatic brain injuries in sports to the attention of the public. Thus far, they have successfully used the media to spread the word about a condition known as chronic traumatic encephalopathy (CTE).[34, 35] A retired professional football player with CTE appeared as a homeless man on a TV episode of *The Gifted Man*. In an episode of the TV series *Harry's Law*, the ethical issues of high school sports' contributions to the growing prevalence of traumatic brain injuries in young athletes was argued by Harry during the case of a young high school football player who died from CTE. While neither of these television shows presented any solutions to the problems of traumatic brain injuries and sports, they were helping to increase a public awareness that "simple blows to the head" do have a long-term impact—especially on young children!

Sadly, there are people among us with other types of severe traumatic brain injuries that are also going unnoticed. They are the veterans who have returned from the Iraq and Afghanistan war with their "Shaken Brain Syndrome"; the Vietnam War Veterans with their own traumatic brain injuries; and the remaining World War II Veterans with their "Shell Shock" injuries.[36, 37] Each group of veterans has their own unique set of symptoms based on the type of warfare employed and the different types of head injuries sustained by the forms of weapons used. In each instance, over time the veteran's external wounds will have healed, yet they are left with invisible injuries that take months to years to heal—if ever! The cognitive changes they recognize can and will become life altering. While they may look normal on the outside, their ability to experience the world has been changed forever. Family and friends do not understand what they are experiencing. Unless the person is left with a physical deformity that others can see and relate to, the world of the veteran with a traumatic brain injury is one that few can comprehend.

The impact of such injuries can be seen in the results from a major 2007–2008 study by the RAND Corporation which demonstrated that 31 percent of the 1.7 million returning soldiers from the Iraq and Afghanistan Wars, or more than 500,000 veterans, will have Post Traumatic Stress Disorder (PTSD), Traumatic Brain Injuries (TBI), and/or depression.[31] Of the 500,000, figures show that as many as 320,000 received traumatic brain injuries. Only half of those with traumatic brain injuries sought treatment for their injuries for fear of being labeled with a mental disorder that could interfere with their military careers. How sad this news is to hear! These men and women are trying to cope with a medical disorder that impacts their cognitive functioning, not a "mental disorder." Specific rehabilitation measures are available to them to help with the adjustments and/or adaptations needed to help them with the changes their brain damage has created. The fallout from their "Shaken Brains" does not have to be the end to their lives in the military nor to their personal lives.

Those veterans from earlier wars are being looked at from different lenses. As these men and women age, their ability to contain the memories and flashbacks created during their war experiences are reduced. Those who fall victim to the neurodegenerative diseases of aging, such as Alzheimer's, are experiencing flashbacks in settings such as nursing homes where their care givers are not skilled or trained to deal with them. Fortunately, some research into the extent of these problems is also being conducted as the issue of long-term effects of head injuries becomes more prominent.

Studies on war veterans and retired professional football players found that both groups were linked to an increased risk for dementia later in life. The veterans who had experienced combat-related head injuries ranging from concussions to severe head wounds were more than twice as likely to develop dementia as their non-brain injury counterparts. Shockingly, 35 percent of the retired football players from the National Football League had signs of dementia. Ongoing research of these two populations continues to add to a growing body of evidence that demonstrates that head injuries of all types can lead to severe long-term consequences many years later. Other athletes being added to these studies include soccer players and swimmers. Like their peers, these athletes are also subject to brain damage from hits to the head. They too face potential long-term consequences from their head traumas.[38]

Clearly there is mounting evidence that many different groups coping with mild, moderate, and/or severe traumatic brain injuries are living with some form of TBI-induced dementia. For those remaining, the likelihood of developing dementia grows over time. As our populations age, we will certainly see more cases emerge.

HIV-AIDS DEMENTIA

With the advances made in the combination antiretroviral therapies (ART) over the past several years, the survival rates for people with HIV-AIDS have improved dramatically.[39] In spite of these advances, HIV-associated neurocognitive disorders (HAND) still create major concerns for health care providers.[40, 41] While they are not universally present in all HIV-infected persons, at least 30 percent of persons with asymptomatic HIV infections and 50 percent of those with acquired immunodeficiency syndrome (AIDS) do exhibit signs and symptoms of some mild neurological disease. It is important to note that the neurocognitive problems associated with an HIV infection are not necessarily progressive. In fact, they may resolve themselves over time with the appropriate treatment regimens.[42]

To receive a diagnosis of HAND, the person must be assessed for at least five areas of neurocognitive functioning that are affected by HIV infections.[43, 44] These include executive functioning, episodic memory, speed of processing information, motor/movement skills, attention and working memory, use of language, and sensori-perception. Due to the high prevalence of other diseases of the central nervous system that are found in the HIV population, making a clear diagnosis of HAND is difficult. Often such a diagnosis rests on determining the presence or absence of the person's self-reported declines in normal everyday functioning as well as other markers associated with the person's medical history.

The growing body of literature on mild neurocognitive declines in HIV-infected persons with no impairment in daily functioning has generated new, more-refined diagnostic distinctions. Asymptomatic neurocognitive impairment (ANI) is the term now being used for this group. These are thought to represent the majority of cases of HAND and 21 to 30 percent of the asymptomatic HIV-infected individuals.[45]

Another term, mild neurocognitive disorder (MND), formerly referred to as MCMD, requires the person to have a mild to moderate neurocognitive impairment in at least two areas of cognitive functioning.[46] A marked decline in activities of daily living that are not linked to co-existing medical conditions or delirium must also be present. Other areas to be considered include unemployment or a reduction in job responsibilities due to reduced cognitive abilities; a decline in vocational functioning as demonstrated by increased errors, decreased productivity, or greater effort needed to perform the work; and/or increased cognitive problems in day-to-day activities.

The most severe form of HAND is HIV-associated dementia (HAD).[47] Having worked with a young man with this condition in the early 1990s, I can attest to the devastation it creates. The criteria for this condition are a moderate to severe decline in cognitive functioning in at least two areas—e.g., language, attention, compre-hension, reasoning, memory, or motor skills—as well as a marked decline in the person's activities of daily living. Unemployment due to cognitive disabilities is included. The young man I worked with had declines in all of the areas mentioned here as well as a host of other problems associated with the other central nervous system diseases that appeared in the final stages of his disease. Fortunately, with the introduction of the combination antiretroviral therapies (ART) in the late 1990s, the prevalence of this condition has been greatly reduced. HIV-AIDS researchers estimate that only 1 to 2 percent of HIV-positive persons meet the criteria for HAD.[48]

An interesting point needs to be made at this juncture. With growing numbers of long-term HIV survivors adding to the aging population comes the problem of HIV-associated Alzheimer's disease. In addition to the Alzheimer's-disease-related risks posed by some of the HIV related complications and treatments, aging long-term HIV survivors will also have a greater vulnerability to common non-HIV pathogens that may contribute to the development of Alzheimer's. The implications of the medical management for long-term HIV patients with chronic dementia are unknown. This area will be fertile territory for future AIDS research.[49]

CHEMOTHERAPY INDUCED DEMENTIA

An even less well-known form of dementia than those already described is the one found among patients who have undergone various types of chemotherapy treatments. "Chemobrain" among women receiving chemotherapy for breast cancer is one example of this condition.[50] Studies of this population in the United States, the Netherlands, Australia, and Canada have all concluded that chemotherapy-induced cognitive dysfunction in these patients does occur.[51, 52, 53, 54, 55] Problems with concentration, memory, attention processes, mental flexibility, speed of information processing, and visual memory have been noted. These cognitive impairments are unaffected by anxiety, depression, fatigue, and time since treatment. Due to a lack of consensus among researchers and medical experts on the exact nature of this form of dementia and its long term clinical presentation, more studies will have to be done to accurately document its full presentation and potential effective treatments.[56, 57]

OPEN HEART SURGERY INDUCED DEMENTIA

Like the dementia associated with chemotherapy, the prevalence of a form of dementia that occurs following open heart procedures has been relatively unknown to the public, though its presence has been noted in the medical literature for many years. With the growing senior population and the increased number of open heart procedures being performed annually, more and more people with this form of dementia are appearing on the health care scene. Currently, some medical experts estimate that as many as 80 percent of all patients undergoing open heart surgery will experience some type of neuropsychological disorder during their post-operative recovery.[58]

Researchers from the United States, Italy, Germany, India, Argentina, and Portugal have all examined the neurocognitive changes that occur after both coronary artery bypass grafting

(CABG) surgeries and heart valve replacement surgeries.[59, 60, 61, 62, 63] Results demonstrate that both short- and long-term cognitive changes do occur, though the exact mechanism by which these changes are produced is not yet understood. It is believed they are multifactorial in nature and not the result of a single event taking place during the surgical procedure. Examples of changes reported by patients and their families include a decline in the patient's memory, problems with mathematical calculations, issues with word fluency, and in some cases, noticeable changes in personality. The growing prevalence of these cognitive changes and others are contributing to neurocognitive dysfunction becoming one of the most frequent complications of cardiac surgery, with documented potential for having a negative impact on the patient's quality of life. Until the mechanisms that produce theses brain changes during open heart surgery are more clearly understood and managed, we can expect to see an increased prevalence of dementia among these aging adults.

♪

While there are many other conditions that can produce dementia, the ones presented here are some of the most common. Reading about even one of them can be exhausting. Becoming knowledgeable about the most prevalent ones is draining. Living with any one of them is life altering.

At this point, I am hopeful that you now understand that dementia comes in many forms. While declines occur in specific areas of cognitive functioning with each of the disorders presented, there are a host of other aspects of intellectual functioning that remain intact and functioning. Accentuating these latter areas will be important for the maintenance of an ongoing quality of life.

♪

Creating the content of this chapter has been extremely challenging. With each disease described comes the face of someone I know/knew and a flood of memories about times we spent together. For most of my life, I have been surrounded by people with some form of dementia—without realizing it! For example, my grandfather, who spent his final years with his seven grandchildren, had multi-infarct dementia. His thwarted speech patterns were "normal" to me. The love he showered all of his grandchildren with during our early years was far more important than his inability to say words correctly. If that were not enough, both of my parents were older adults when my sisters and I were born. My father, who was nearing retirement age when I was still in elementary school, was already showing some aspects of a "normal aging memory decline!" The fact that he was my father was far more important to me than his ability to remember specific details of daily life.

The number of people with dementias brought on by Alzheimer's disease, Huntington's disease, Parkinson's disease, post chemotherapy treatments, post open heart procedures, traumatic brain injuries, war-related traumas, athletic injuries sustained by anyone from high school heroes to major professional athletes, and HIV are overwhelming. Over my forty years of working in the healthcare industry, many of them have crossed my path. Their faces and their individual stories have flooded my mind as I worked diligently to give you some idea of the challenges their medical problems created. It is their stories and those challenges they have faced each day that led to the creation of this chapter. It is important for everyone to have a basic understanding of what dementia is and what is not. As the number of people with some form of a dementia process continues to increase over the coming decades, we as a society may be a bit better prepared to work with them if we have some understanding of what they are experiencing.

A picture of Helga Rohra's term "dementia consciousness" is becoming more clear in my mind. With the growing numbers of aging adults around the world who will likely develop some form of dementia, we are going to be faced with its impact on our lives. Everyone will know about dementia. Dementia will become part of our everyday language. In many places, women and men with dementia will be living alone.[64] We will be forced to change our perspective on how we treat these individuals. Realizing each person still has existing abilities will be the first step. Promoting those abilities will be the next step. Adapting to any weaknesses that occur in the person as the dementia process changes over time will also be necessary.

Efforts will have to be made to adapt to this phenomena as it spreads. These people have assets that make them valuable to the members of their immediate community. They have lessons to teach us all about aging and the diseases that rob us of some—but not all—of our intellectual abilities. Even those with profound dementias—as seen in end-stage Alzheimer's—have contributions to make to our lives *if* we allow them.

As I have noted, creating and maintaining connections with these individuals is important. It is something that must be learned. It is not hard. It takes time and some patience but once learned becomes second nature. Rewards are awaiting those who are willing to learn just how to establish these connections. In the coming pages,

I will talk about spirituality and the human spirit. Learning how to make a connection to the human spirit of a person with dementia is the first step. Once this connection has been established, the next step is to open a door to the person's memories. In the pages that follow this second step will come descriptions of several ways to tap a dementia patient's memories.

THREE

A Path to the Inner World of Dementia

The most beautiful things cannot be seen or touched.
They must be felt with the heart.

—Helen Keller

Although dementia will manifest itself differently across people, places and diseases, there is one common thread that runs through all of the people. That thread is the person's "human spirit." Every person has one. It is that "essence" that gives life to each of us. It is alive and functioning. We know there are a plethora of diseases that abound in this world, and any one of them can ravage the human body over time—even the simple process of aging. Ironically, though, none of them can touch the human spirit that still resides inside. It is this spirit that provides a conduit to the inner world of dementia.

Until someone creates a new term for addressing "the domain of the spirit," we are called upon to use the term "spirituality." When the topic of spirituality comes up in a conversation, many people roll their eyes and turn away. Why? There are so many different views of just what spirituality means. No two people ever seem to be on the same page when they are talking about spirituality.

Many years ago, I began researching the topic of spirituality for a presentation I was making to a group of American health care professionals at their annual convention. I thought the task of finding a common definition for it would be easy. I naively thought that if I did the proper research, I could uncover a definition that would be comprehensive enough for everyone to agree upon. After days of reviewing definition after definition from page after page of reference materials, I became totally overwhelmed and gave up. It appeared that everyone had his or her own definition of spirituality! How was I going to make a presentation on spirituality and its relationship to health if I could not provide a clear definition that could work for the majority of people in the audience?

Anyone who has ever heard me give a speech on the subject knows that I finally came upon a definition that is broad enough to allow anyone to take it and work with it. Indeed, the definition I use *is* broad. It is open to one's interpretation, and it can be incorporated into anyone's personal belief system. Over time I came to understand that each person's view of "spirituality" is based on that individual's personal background and life experiences, religious training (if any), and/or a belief system about the "essence" that gives us life. Beyond any of these, it is the experiences one has over a lifetime that shape the individual's views and understanding of what spirituality and the human spirit mean *to them*. Many people around the world have told me about events they have had at one time or another that *had no rational explanations*. Like them, I had also witnessed events that were extraordinary. As I mentioned earlier in this book, while I was in the midst of having a motor vehicle accident, I heard voices say "you will

THREE: A PATH TO THE INNER WORLD OF DEMENTIA

not die." I looked in the direction of the voices. There was no one there. Next, these same voices told me to "lean into the door." I complied. This *extraordinary* experience probably saved my life.

Like the others who told me about their *extraordinary* encounters *I had no rational or logical explanation for any of theirs or mine.* Because I am a trained scientist, none of these experiences set well with my rational mind or my linear form of thinking. I knew that I was not crazy in any sense of the word, but I needed some cogent explanations for what I had heard, seen, and experienced. After all, I had to live with mine as well as theirs and move on with my own life.

Over time, I came to realize that *spirituality* and *religiousness* do hold the same meanings for me that many others have. Anyone who has read *Symphony of Spirits* is familiar with my background: my Southern Protestant religious upbringing and my Catholic nursing school training. For me it has become more and more important to make a distinction between the world of "spirit" and the world of "religion." The following definitions offered many years ago by a group of well-respected researchers helped me. By reading them, you may begin to understand the distinction I make between these two very different worlds:

> *Religiousness…has specific behavioral, societal, doctrinal and denominational characteristics because it involves a system of worship and doctrine that is shared within a group.*
>
> *Spirituality is concerned with the transcendent, addressing ultimate questions about life's meaning, with the assumption that there is more to life than what we see or fully understand. It can call us beyond self to concern and compassion for others.*[65]

The definition of spirituality that I give to people in my public presentations was offered many years ago by a well-respected psychiatrist, Dr. C. Kuhn. "Spirituality", he said, "...are those capacities that enable a human being to rise above or transcend any experience at hand. They are characterized by the capacity to seek meaning and purpose, to have faith, to love, to forgive, to pray, to meditate, to worship, and to see beyond the present circumstances."[66] Those capacities are found in the human spirit. And what is the human spirit? For me, it is the vital essence of a person, the principle of life—commonly regarded as an entity distinct from the body, or as some understand it, the human soul. It helps that person to understand events that occur in his or her life that defy all logical and/or scientific explanations. When it comes to working around persons with dementia, one must *be able to think in terms of the human spirit as a distinct entity* that is separate from the flesh and blood body the outside world recognizes. *This entity is a separate component of the individual and always remains untouched by those illnesses and traumas that alter the functioning of that person's physical body.*[67] If you can wrap your head around this concept, you can begin to recognize that a part of the dementia-stricken loved one remains present and ready for interacting with the outside world.

It took many weeks and months for me to begin to understand this concept. It was originally taught to me by three women with various Native American orientations to the spirit world. Consequently, I don't expect a novice to the world of spirits, spirituality, or soul communications to grasp it immediately. It took a trip to an Elisabeth Kübler-Ross Life, Death, and Transition (LDT) workshop for me to even begin to comprehend this approach to dementia care.[68, 69]

The LDT was one of a four-part series of workshops on how to cope with death and dying that Dr. Kübler-Ross and her staff taught in various parts of the world. I would soon come to learn that it also

THREE: A PATH TO THE INNER WORLD OF DEMENTIA

offered participants a different perspective on how to cope with losses of all types. My LDT classmates and I were fortunate enough to receive personal lessons from Dr. Kübler-Ross herself, whose groundbreaking book *On Death and Dying* had brought her world-wide recognition. The book remains the gold standard of the world's hospice movement, and her five stages of death and dying have become a part of the standard nomenclature for the grieving process. The following excerpt from *Symphony of Spirits* on my experiences at this very important workshop may offer a better perspective on spirituality for those who need a more concrete explanation:

> *The workshop program was stunning and unlike anything I had encountered in my years of formal medical training. The small-group discussions that followed the structured educational sessions exposed me to an entirely new view of the death-and-dying process.*
>
> *For one intensive week, I was closely associated with professional men and women from medicine, business, and philanthropic agencies who were not afraid to question the ironclad rules of science and medicine. In fact, many of the participants were boldly challenging the accepted orthodoxy because of unexplainable things from their own experiences with dying patients, clients, friends, and relatives. Many members of my seminar class were veteran health workers with thousands of combined hours of experienced gained in cancer hospices and other centers dedicated to assisting dying patients.*
>
> *Most important for me, however, was the fact that by participating in the academically approved seminar, I had been exposed to physicians, nurses, hospice workers, grief counselors, and other professionals who were looking at nontraditional approaches to dealing with death and dying.*

It was as if I had been given some official stamp of approval to examine the alternatives.

The centerpiece of the LDT workshop was Dr. Kübler-Ross's Four-Quadrant Theory of Personality Development. Each of the four quadrants—the physical, the emotional, the intellectual, and the spiritual—addresses a different aspect of personality. Dr. Kübler-Ross taught that development accelerates in the spiritual quadrant as a person moves closer to death.

The fact that this noted physician espoused a similar theory of spiritual development in the fourth quadrant supported some of the contentions being made by my new nurse friends...who insisted that they could see the spirits of patients with advanced dementia more clearly than those of other elderly patients with intact thinking and remembering abilities. Since these old people were closer to death, their spirit images were stronger. And since their earthly mental process were suspended by their disease, their spirit natures were the only thing functioning strongly with them.

The goal of applying the Kübler-Ross quadrant theoretical model is not as all-encompassing as the (Native American) shaman teachings. The model was part of an instructional tool used by Dr. Kübler-Ross and her staff to teach people about how and when in life we learn to grieve a loss. Kübler-Ross's theory suggests that there are four basic stages of human development. The stages begin at different ages in a person's life and continue to develop and overlap until death. Since the quadrants are depicted in a circle—a circle divided into four parts—it also suggests a continuation of the life cycle beyond human existence into a spiritual dimension.

Three: A Path to the Inner World of Dementia

The <u>physical quadrant</u> begins at birth and includes the development of the human body as well as the five senses: sight, hearing, smell, taste, and touch. Human beings and all higher animals are born into the world with the basic tools for these, including the obvious: eyes for sight, ears for hearing, nose and tongue for smell and taste. The sense of touch or feeling is a bit more complicated but, likewise, is attributed to physical nerve networks. For example, nerve endings in the skin convey sensations of heat, cold, pressure, or pain.

Physical development also includes the functioning of internal organs, such as the heart, stomach, and nerves, which govern such sensations as fatigue, hunger and thirst, and balance. In each instance, the features of the physical quadrant are well known to us and quantifiable by accepted medical testing procedures.

If it all ended right there, the explanation of life would be far less complicated, and we would be pretty much like all the other living creatures on Earth, from bugs to bison. If this were all there was to life, I could have labored happily in surgical nursing for the rest of my days, since modern medicine has become proficient at patching up the physical body and even replacing failing organs.

But at about the age of six months, humans begin to develop another characteristic, represented by the <u>emotional quadrant.</u> Relationships are formed from a need to love and be loved. When these needs for love go unfulfilled, the person ceases to develop normally, resulting in feelings of rejection, abandonment, and betrayal. Development in this quadrant can be identified, if not exactly measured, by a person's behavior and ability to deal with other people.

At about the age of six (experts differ widely on when this phase begins in the young child), development begins in the <u>intellectual quadrant</u>. This is the period of time when there is the recognition of a "need to know" and when the child begins to exercise some logic. Obviously, if this phase of development is not fully realized, the person becomes what some refer to as "intellectually challenged," and human potential goes unmet. In this developmental quadrant, intellect can be measured to some degree by standard testing systems, such as Intelligence Quotient (IQ) tests.

Spiritual development, represented by the <u>spiritual quadrant</u>, begins in adolescence, according to Dr. Kübler-Ross. Development continues throughout life in all quadrants. However, the spiritual aspect actually becomes more intense as a person ages. Of course, spiritual development is the most difficult area to measure quantitatively or define in any scientific sense. Thus, science and medicine largely choose to ignore this aspect of humanity. Failure to develop human spirituality can be observed in some people as confusion or an aura of emptiness and in others as a lost sense of purpose in life and a strong fear of death.

...Dr. Kübler-Ross taught that death was simply a transition process in which the soul or spirit moves from this world to the next. She stressed that a person's spiritual quadrant actually becomes more intense as the person ages. Such ideas coming from one of the world's most respected thanatologists helped to add a level of confidence to my growing belief in the existence of a spirit realm and an afterlife.

With Dr. Kübler-Ross's passing a few years ago, her well trained staff continues her work. They offer workshops based on her

Three: A Path to the Inner World of Dementia

teachings for those who are trying to cope with grief issues (www.externalizationworkshops.com). Knowing their outreach is limited to people who are fortunate enough to learn about their offerings, I was pleased to find someone taking up the banner on spirituality in a much different way—the United States Military!

With the growing number of men and women soldiers returning from the Iraq and Afghanistan wars with multiple physical and psychological issues, it appears that some of their leaders are making an effort to address the "spiritual fitness in the Army."[70] According to two authors who write about this topic, K.I. Pargament and P.J. Sweeney, the Army has identified spirituality as a salient dimension of its strategic planning and training programs.[71] Finally! I mention this work for the sole purpose of letting readers know that even the US Military has now acknowledged the importance of addressing the spiritual dimension of its soldiers.

Within the US Army's New Comprehensive Soldier Fitness Program, spirituality is defined in the human sense as "the journey people take to discover and realize their essential selves and higher order aspirations."[72] It is a necessary component of this new program because Army leaders believe that it is "a significant motivating force – a vital resource for human development and a source of struggle for many soldiers." They address spirituality in the human sense rather than in a theological sense. For this I am grateful. I only hope that it allows persons involved in the program to incorporate the material on spirituality in a manner that fits their own personal belief systems.

The Department of Defense, according to Pargament and Sweeney, is trying to facilitate the search for truth, self-knowledge, purpose, and direction in life among its soldiers. Within this new program, "spirit" is further defined as "the essential core of the individual, the deepest part of the self and one's evolving human essence.... [I]t is thoroughly manifested in who we are." It is not the same as one's personal identity. It helps individuals organize their lives and move themselves forward.[73]

For these same leaders "spirituality" refers to "the continuous journey people take to discover and realize their spirit—that is—their essential selves.... [S]pirituality is the process of searching for the sacred in one's life. From this developmental perspective, people can take any variety of pathways in an effort to develop the human spirit. Nature, music, exercise, loving relationships, scientific exploration, religion, work, art, philosophy, and study are just a few of the paths that people follow in their efforts to grow spiritually."[74]

From these words, it appears that the US Military leaders are following a developmental approach to spirituality similar to the one Dr. Kübler-Ross laid out decades earlier. Why do I bother taking readers down this path? Dr. Kübler-Ross and the US Military leaders are worlds apart in the grand scheme of life, yet they both arrived at similar understandings of what spirituality means to many people! There must be something to this approach—if nothing more than its ability to provide people with a definition of spirituality they can wrap their heads around.

Spending so much time on formulating a cogent and precise definition of what spirituality means is important. Why? Creating connections with another person through the dimension known as "spirit" can open doorways—doorways to a type of communication process that persons with dementia can "hear." To accomplish this very important feat, one *must* have a working idea of what "the human spirit" is and what "spirituality" means.

Now what do I mean by "persons with dementia can hear"? We are told by experts that persons with different types of dementias cannot

Three: A Path to the Inner World of Dementia

recognize the world around them nor the people in it. How can they "hear anything"? How can they make meaning of it? Many years ago, as I have mentioned earlier, a Cherokee elder told me the "heart has ears." The heart can "hear." "Speak to the heart and the spirit will hear what is being said," he told me.[75] It made sense to me. I had seen this happen with many of the people I worked with over the years—persons with different stages of Alzheimer's dementia as well as other illnesses that created a form of dementia.

Soon after my encounter with the Cherokee elder, I met a very interesting woman who studies Egyptian hieroglyphics, Normandy Ellis. Normandy leads tours to Egypt and writes extensively about her knowledge of the Egyptian history acquired from years of study. In her book *Awakening Osiris: The Egyptian Book of the Dead*, Normandy offered some very interesting information about the views of the spiritual world during earlier times based on her translations of two-thousand-year-old hieroglyphics.[76] According to Egyptian theology, she writes, "the structure of a man is not limited only to his mortal shell and spiritual self, but it is a complex and interconnected structure where his physical body, spiritual body, mental and emotional states play on each other."[77] Does any of this sound familiar? She goes on to say that the term *ab* "is the heart, the seat of knowledge, wisdom and understanding; it is the link between the physical body and the spiritual body.... Ab represents what a man may come to know of the world and himself in silent meditation."[78] For anyone who wishes to learn more about Egyptian spirituality, she recommends reading John West's *Serpent in the Sky* and several books by R. A. Schwaller de Lubicz and his wife, Isha, including *Opening the Way, Symbol and the Symbolic, Nature Word,* and *The Temple of Man*.

For more than a decade, I worked with people at this "spirit level." I talked to their spirit in "one-way conversations" each time I was near them. In other words, I would initiate a normal conversation with a dementia patient. The topics would vary from what I saw outside their window, to what I was about to do with them, to the how they looked at that moment. They never gave me a response. I never expected one. The conversation was going one-way – from me to them. I made an assumption that their spirit could hear my words and my message. Little did I know at the time that I was working within a realm of life that was known to many other cultures for centuries!

As I mentioned earlier, only recently was I given a new and improved way to understand what was happening in these one-way conversations. While attending a conference in Atlanta where the Dalai Lama and several medical researchers from across the country discussed the biological basis for compassion, I heard a piece of information that explained this "heart-spirit-mind" connection. One of the presenters from the University of North Carolina, Dr. Barbara Frederickson, and her colleagues described how the vagal nerve carries information from the brain to the heart and back again.[79, 80] Dr. Frederickson's research has centered on this connection and how it contributes to an understanding of the biological foundation for compassion. For me, it identified an open biological-sensory channel available for the human spirit to transport information from the heart to the head! Speaking directly to a dementia person's heart sets up a sensory-vibrational wave transmission process that carries information from the heart to the brain and back to the heart via the vagus nerve (the tenth cranial nerve)! This neural connection in the brain then sets off other neural activities within the human body! Now, this may be a stretch for many people, but for me it gave new meaning to the phrase "the heart can hear."

The researchers at the Dali Lama's conference were describing one of the biological pathways for the popular phrase "mind-body" connection. While there are many other biological, psychological, and medical intricacies to the mind-body connection, this basic piece of information serves my purpose. It establishes a foundation for understanding the material that will follow.

There are many different avenues through which anyone can make connections with a person who is living with a dementia process. They are simple, concrete, and effective. One must keep in mind that each time one of these avenues is traveled, it will "touch the spirit" of the person with dementia in some way. The interaction can be helpful and healing for both people! I have seen it happen.

FOUR

Soul Strings

It is only with the heart that one can see rightly what is essential is invisible to the eye.

—from *The Little Prince*
by Antoine de Saint-Exupéry

Making connections to the inner world of a person with dementia is easier than most people realize. Dr. Thomas Moore, noted author of *Care for the Soul,* points out that "anyone can make connections to the human soul by simply asking questions. Inquiries about the person's early life, childhood activities, past loves, family members, favorite pets, or even work-related accomplishments can open pathways to old memories and establish connections to a host of pathways. The use of sensual language can often help trigger pleasant memories.."[81]

MUSIC

There are a host of other ways to establish connections beyond making simple inquires about a person's past—especially for those who have issues with speech generation. The first one that people seem to grasp easily is the use of music. Regardless of one's age or circumstances, there is always some genre of music that seems to strike a chord in the heart and soul of the listener. My very first experience with this phenomenon came with a group of profoundly demented people sitting together in a day room listening to a videotape of different choirs singing *Amazing Grace.* Regardless of their stage of dementia progression, each person "heard" the music. Their responses were as different as their diseases. Some began singing along. Others were rocking back and forth in their seats. Still others could do nothing more than tap their foot on the floor to the rhythm of the sounds. But they were all smiling. It was amazing to watch.

An even more profound example of music's impact on a person with dementia is a story I was told about an elderly man in a nursing home in North Carolina. According to one of the ladies who was present there that day, a staff member sat down at an old upright piano in the day room and began to play the song *Amazing Grace.* Upon hearing the sounds of music, many of the patients on the unit as well as other staff members began to gather around the piano. Soon everyone began to sing along—except for an old man slumped over in a chair in the corner of the room.

Everyone thought the old man could not speak. He had not uttered a word to anyone in years. Each day a staff member would have to bring him into the day room in a wheelchair. His frail body was then transferred to the same chair in the same corner of the day room. He would remain there for most of the day until someone came to retrieve him and return him to his room.

On this particular day, something very strange happened. As the piano's chords sent music out and across the room, the voices of those singing along added to the volume of the soulful sounds. No one was paying attention to the old man; they were all caught up in the moment. Suddenly, the old man stood up! Still no one noticed him. As he walked across the room toward the piano unassisted by anyone, the silence that swept across the room was deafening. The old man walked over to the piano on his own power. He propped his right arm on top of the old upright piano, and he began to sing. Soon the others—still in shock—joined him. Over the next several minutes, the old man smiled as he stared at the ceiling and sang every word to every verse of *Amazing Grace*. When the song was over and the music stopped, the old man quietly removed his arm from the top of the piano and walked slowly back to his familiar chair in the corner of the room. He sat down in the chair and never uttered another word!

Amazing Grace is a song familiar to many elderly people who are currently in their 80s, 90s, and 100s. They grew up hearing it. It was a part of the fabric of their lives. With subsequent generations that follow this one, there will be other songs that resonate to them. Those songs will be a part of their unique generational histories. For some it will be the sounds of the big bands, swing music, the jitterbug, bee bop, or the early days of the Grand Ole Opry—people like Mother May Bell Carter and the Carter Family. Others will come alive to the sounds of people like Judy Garland, Johnny Mathis, Tony Bennett, Jerry Lee Lewis, or some of the more contemporary Old World classics like Rachmaninoff. For others it will be the sounds of Elvis Presley and the rock and roll era of Aretha Franklin, Otis Redding, Gladys Night and the Pips, the Monkeys, The Beach Boys, Glen Campbell, Kenny Rogers, The Rolling Stones, Rod Stewart, Ike & Tina Turner, the Beatles, or Michael Jackson that will get their feet tapping and their heads swaying. Still others' eyes will show signs of life when they hear the soulful sounds of Miles Davis and other great musicians of jazz.

When I ask people of my generation what song will ring true to their souls, the answer is always without hesitation "Stairway to Heaven"! Unless a cure for Alzheimer's disease and the many other conditions that can produce dementia is found, we can expect that the current crop of young people will find their aging bodies reverberating to the current sounds of people like Eminem, Jay Z, Beyoncé, Lady Gaga, Adele, Tupac, Usher, Justin Beiber, and hip hop moguls of the new millennium! Can you even imagine what that will look like?

Such stories should make us stop to think about the power of music and its importance to the developing brains of our children. Music and the arts lay solid foundations for a unique growth process in the brains of children everywhere—a foundation that can serve them well into their later years of life! Support for this idea comes from several well-respected medical specialists, such as Dr. Oliver Sacks, Professor of Neurology and Psychiatry at Columbia University and noted author of such popular books as *The Man Who Mistook his Wife for a Hat, Awakenings*, and *Musicophilia: Tales of Music and the Brain*; therapeutic musician Barbara Jacobs, who produced a series of music sing-along DVDs for Alzheimer's patients and seniors; Kim Watkins, an executive program director at an acquired brain injury rehabilitation center; and Dr. Daniel Levitin, an associate professor at the University of California–Davis Center for Mind and Brain.[82, 83, 84, 85]

Dr. Sacks notes that everyone with any form of dementia—without exception—will respond to music. This is especially true of old songs from their early life and old songs they once knew. Music appears to touch threads of emotion and memory which are inaccessible in any other way. It seems to trigger old memories of when the person heard that particular song! That sort of lucidity and pleasure, Dr. Sacks points out, can last for hours after the song has ended.

Personal memories are embedded in emotional responses. Dr. Daniel Levitin, author of *This is Your Brain on Music*, points out that people "remember things that have an emotional component because our amygdala (a critical part of the brain for emotional responses) and neurotransmitters act in concert to tag as important the memories of these emotionally charged years of self-discovery." According to researchers in this area, these years are the teen years. At around the age of fourteen, people's musical preferences and memories are formed.[86] With the ongoing trend of the music industry to get music to younger and younger children, I suspect this data may be revised at some point in the future. Regardless of what the ongoing research is telling us at this point in history, we know from well-documented sources that people with dementia of the Alzheimer's type, as well as those with other forms of dementia, can often sing songs they heard in their teen years—even when they cannot remember the names of their own family members!

Researchers like Petr Janata, associate professor at the University of California–Davis Center for Mind and Brain, are actively conducting research on the human brain's response to music. In time, he and others are hoping to develop music-based therapies for persons with dementia. For now there are centers around the globe that are creating their own music therapy programs that tap into the music of their culture, like those in India, Brazil, Argentina, Chile, Bulgaria, Croatia, Germany, and China. Some of those programs, like the one Kim Watkins described in her work with acquired brain injury patients in the USA, use some of the simplest musical items that are available to anyone. Things like a toy holiday doll that plays familiar Christmas songs over and over again or an old CD of songs by a familiar artist have meaning to people. They tap old memories. They put smiles on people's faces. They can bring joy to a world of emptiness. They can even make a dark, lonely room seem less confusing.[87] The power of music is truly awesome.

EXPRESSION THROUGH PAINTING AND DRAWING

Music is not the only form of art that can open a door to the inner world of dementia. During a visit to a Texas Alzheimer's Association office several years ago, I was given the privilege of touring a collection of art works created by Alzheimer's patients. Each piece was filled with vibrant colors. The images seemed to be saying: "there is still a person in here." If there is any question about this observation, take a look at some of the beautiful artwork used by many Alzheimer's chapters in their annual fundraising calendars.

In Northern California there are art programs available in several communities that are designed specifically for persons with various forms of dementia, not just Alzheimer's.[88] Their goal is to give these people a way to express themselves when they are having trouble finding words or even saying anything. The participants range from former artists to people who have never held a paintbrush. The organizers point out that the program provides a valuable tool for communication and memory retrieval and for boosting the participant's confidence.

In the quiet rooms where the art classes take place, art supplies are provided. Watercolors seem to be the easiest to work with. Instructors are available to help each person get started on a painting. Stories abound of people in their eighties and nineties who discover they have a talent for drawing or painting. Likewise, many family members are surprised and shocked by what they see. A line of communication may open up that was not available. Often while painting, participants see an image that triggers a memory and words suddenly rush out. In this low-stress environment, it is the process not the product that is important. It is the discovery of what comes from the "process of painting" that is valued.[88]

The act of drawing or painting is not the only way persons with any form of dementia can utilize art. In cities like Ft. Worth, Texas, and New York City, art museums are creating programs for people with dementias to come and spend time viewing well-known paintings, sculptures, and other pieces of art. Why? Like music, the images in the paintings or sculptures trigger memories inside the person. Those memories are attached to words that often find their way out of the fog that is created by a dementia process. Conversations begin. Sharing takes place. For a while there is a connection to the outside world and to others. Everyone is alive in the moment there in the museum.[89]

REMINISCENCE THERAPY

Reminiscence therapy is popular among nursing homes across the United States. It is simple for most staff members to use with patients who are in varying stages of progressive dementias. The goal of this therapy is the get patients to reminisce and talk about earlier times. It is designed to stimulate long term memories. Sadly, I have never seen it produce useful results in groups where very demented persons are present and disruptive to the group process. When it is done in settings where family members are present and interested in the family histories that can be shared, this type of therapy can be very rewarding.

While attending a recent concert of the legendary singer Aretha Franklin, I was inspired by Mr. Robinson, a handsome young gentleman who was assigned the task of "warming up" the audience. He began his routine with "back in the day" stories. When he mentioned the days of white bread and fried bologna sandwiches, I was hooked. Being raised in the South, I knew all too well what he was describing. Next there was a reference to the government cheese! Every child who attended grammar school "back in the day" can remember the big blocks of government cheese provided to lunch rooms across the South.

Children at school were fed nourishing meals by women who knew how to use local foods and government food subsidies to create meals we wanted to eat. As he reminded us that night, "back in the day" no one went hungry! We all took care of each other and shared what we had! When the stories about Kool-Aid and the simple television shows from the 1950s came around, I was transported to another time.

Maybe we should drop reminiscence therapy and start having "back in the day" conversations with our elders. When Dr. Thomas Moore suggested that we use "sensual language" to access the soul, I thought immediately about sex. After hearing Mr. Robinson's descriptions of life "back in the day," I realized that "sensual language" can have many meanings. When talk of a fried bologna sandwich and a glass of ice-cold Kool-Aid on a hot summer's day came around, I could feel my mouth water and the back of my neck begin to sweat! For a moment, I was seven years old riding my bicycle down an old country road! Images of "back in the day" can be filled with so many memories. It conjures up mental pictures in all of us.

STORYTELLING

When someone starts talking about life "back in the day," memories are jogged to the forefront of your mind. Stories spring forth from that "well of memories" that usually remains silent. One story begets another. When this happens some people are wise enough to drag out an audiotape recorder and capture the moments of memories shared. Others who are more fortunate will grab a video camera or cell phone camera and create a piece of family history. Time and again, I have had family members tell me how grateful they were to have images and sounds of a loved one available to them long after that person has passed on.

MAKING FRIENDS WITH THE ENEMY

While I was in graduate school and working on a geriatric unit, my Native American nurse friends spent hours teaching me about the spiritual aspects of a dementia process. I struggled with the information they were sharing with me. All of them knew that I did not want to be working on that dementia unit.. I needed the money, and it was the best job for me to have at the time. Time and again they would watch as the patients on our unit would begin to display their daily "sundowning process." It always got to me. Two or more people would start screaming in the mid-afternoon just as I tried to finish my afternoon assignments. This mayhem would quickly spread across the unit. Other patients sitting in the dayroom would start making single repetitive sounds—echolalia at its highest, most irritating point. Soon the entire unit was filled with sounds that would not stop, no matter what anyone did to abate the noise level.

"Deborah, you are going to have to make friends with this place or it will eat you alive," Ms. Dolly said to me one day.[90]

"What are you talking about?" I replied with a complete look of confusion.

"Emotions have power. Anger is a very powerful emotion. As long as you hang on to your anger about working here, *it—the anger—will hold its power over you*," she replied. "It will control you every day. It will rob you of everything you have, or think you have. You have to make friends with the anger and the situation that is causing it. Only then will it lose its power over you! Only then will you be in control of your world!"

For a long time, her words were puzzling to me. How could I master such a task? How could I put a stop to getting angry every afternoon when those awful screeching sounds began to stream across the room? Let me assure you that it took weeks of thought and soul searching for me to find the answers to these puzzling questions for myself. Next, I had to learn that every person has to find the answers to these same questions on her own.

Learning to let go of my anger started with examining the memories those screeching sounds triggered in me and addressing the learned responses that I had maintained for decades. Once I was able to understand what was happening and make peace with it, I was able to let go of the anger. Trust me: That process took a very long time. My early goals in life did not include nursing. Nursing was the profession my parents chose for me. At the time, there was federal funding for nursing school. Over time, I adapted to the demands of hospital nursing. It gave me money and some freedoms, but it never gave me the happiness that people feel when they are doing a job they enjoy. At this point in my life, I was finally making progress toward a new career that would give me more freedom to use my talents and skills. I felt frustrated and helpless that I had to continue working as a nurse in a place that so unpleasant to me. My enemies were past life events that seemed to have been controlling my life. Eventually, I was able to make peace with those enemies! The "enemies" that generated the anger came from inside of me. Once I able to recognize them, I realized that I had choices about how to respond to them. *I could decide how I was going to react to them.* After weeks of practice, I realized that I had *finally* regained my own power! The sounds of the patients sun-downing did not bother me.

As simple as this little exercise sounds, it was anything but simple. Many people never figure out how to do it. In the world of dementia, this can be a major problem for everyone. Anger abounds for so many. One very powerful way to deal with this anger is by getting it out into the open. Deal with it in a constructive way. Create win-win situations.

HEART-TO-HEART CONVERSATIONS

In heart-to-heart conversations, a heart-felt message is spoken by one person to another. For those individuals with intact cognitive processes, these conversations can be a two-way event. For those who no longer possess any measure of memory, these conversations will be one-way. The gift of profound dementia, especially in the Alzheimer's type, is that nothing said to the person will be registered in that person's physical memory bank. It will be "remembered" in the soul's registry of life events.

What does one discuss in heart-to-heart conversations? For those individuals who only have a short time remaining with the loved one, it is the "unfinished business" between the two. This can mean an open and unedited expression or discussion of memories about earlier events in life that did not get addressed, hurt feelings that have lingered for years, and untold secrets that were never shared. It can be as simple as saying "I love you." Keep in mind that these heart-to-heart conversations are usually for the person speaking, not the person with the dementia. The receiver may smile or stare blankly into space as each emotionally laden phrase comes pouring out. Something very strange happens after heart-to-heart conversations have taken place. Once the air has been cleared, words expressed, emotions released, tears shed, memories released, a change is the relationship between these two people invariably takes place. Everything that needs to be said has been spoken. There is no unfinished business between the two people. The relationship is transformed. I have heard people from all parts of the world tell me this fact For those who have a dementia process that allows some of their cognitive processes to remain intact, these heart-to-heart conversations will cover different material. The topics will vary by person and by events. For those with traumatically induced head injuries, the emotional responses may be out of character or driven by injured brain tissue. For those with a dementia process that is caused by other diseases, the responses can be equally varied. Regardless of the cause for the dementia process, the goal of heart-to-heart conversations is to have honest and forthright expressions of emotions that are healing for both parties and their relationship. Keep in mind that these types of conversations may occur during other venues: while gardening, participating in an art class, playing a board game, putting together a jigsaw puzzle, or simply sitting together watching TV. There is no one place that is better than another. The bottom line is this: They need to happen.

POETRY

One afternoon while I was sitting in a bookstore having tea, a plump, rather plainly dressed middle-aged woman sat down next to me. We began to talk. When I explained to her my reasons for being in the area, a big smile instantly spread across her face. She told me that she was a retired Catholic nun. At the time of our meeting, she was working as a sitter for a very well-heeled woman who was in the latter stages of Alzheimer's disease. The woman no longer spoke. The retired nun said that she was always looking for ways to engage the woman during the hours they were together. Without missing a beat, she began to share this story:

One afternoon the sitter began to read from a book of poetry. The book was one of her favorites. She imagined that at least for that afternoon, she could function in her duties as a sitter and still do something that was enjoyable for her. Suddenly, the old woman began to recite the words to each verse of poetry the sitter read aloud. The retired nun was shocked. She had never even heard the old woman speak. Soon the woman was reciting the words to each verse of the poem—from memory. It seems this stately woman of means had enjoyed poetry in her earlier years.

As she told me this story, this gentle woman's saintly-looking face lit up. She was excited to find something the two women could share. Every afternoon the two would sit for hours reading and reciting poetry. As I listened to this story, I began to think about other ways to make such impactful connections with that inner world of dementia. I came up with the use of music, poetry, working in the garden, playing board games, simple conversations between two people, telling stories to others, and reminiscing sessions. Surely there are more pathways. My quest to find as many pathways as possible to the inner world of a person's dementia began that day!

CREATIVE CUING (STIMULATING) ENVIRONMENTS

One day, a very excited nursing assistant from a local senior center in Oregon came up to me after a presentation to her state organization. She wanted to tell me what she and her co-workers had done to help their residents. Each resident's family was questioned about the early life of that person. What type of work did he or she do over the years?

What had been their daily routine? With this information in hand, this young woman and her co-workers set about creating each resident's room with decorations, designs, and images that had meaning to that individual. She reminded me that the residents in her work setting all were living with some form of dementia, mostly Alzheimer's.

She beamed as she described the unique settings that were created for each of the residents. For the barber, they had placed an old-time red, white, and blue striped barber pole on the wall beside the door that led to his room. Next to it, they painted the image of a window that looked into the barber shop. For the mailman residing on the unit, the staff placed an actual mailbox on a post outside of his door. The wall outside of his room was painted to resemble a post office. When he received mail from the outside world, it went into his personal mailbox. One lady whose life had centered on the flower boxes in front of her house and her flower gardens was given images of flower boxes on the walls outside of her room. The stories went on and on about how each resident had the walls and doorway to their room decorated with images that had meaning just for them.

Finally, after she had described the last room, this young woman looked at me with pride in her eyes. She began to tell me about some of the unexpected behaviors they witnessed. After going to such unusual lengths to make each resident feel "at home," the staff discovered that the residents—with varying stages of dementia—no longer got lost. Rather than wandering about trying to figure out where they were and what was happening around them, each day they went straight to and from their own rooms every time. They were less anxious and more at ease. They responded to images they could see and recognize from another time in their lives—like the man with the striped barber pole on the wall outside of his room. Even the families of these residents enjoyed coming to visit. The environment was alive with images of life. On some units, the images on the walls gave the appearance of a small main street from years gone by.

SAFE HAVENS

The preceding story of what one group of people did to improve the lives of their charges with dementia brings home a very important feature of dementia that most people do not address: a sense of safety! Creating this sense of safety is critical to the person whose cognitive abilities are altered either temporarily or permanently. I cannot begin to explain the depths of fear that come with the loss of any of one's cognitive abilities, whether from a traumatic brain injury or from the slow and progressive loss of an awareness of one's environment that comes with Alzheimer's or any one of the other diseases that I have already mentioned. Sounds of all types are exaggerated—painfully in some instances! Images don't always make sense. Watching a friend's lips move and not understanding the words and sounds that come out can be devastating. Being trapped in a body that no longer works the way it did yesterday or last week or last year is confusing and terrifying.

Familiar faces bring some relief and comfort. Sadly, though, they do not quell the panic attacks that can spring up from being left alone in a strange place. Nor does their presence suppress the volleys of rage that can erupt from the slightest comment uttered in the room. A loss of coherent speech can be frightening. Opening one's mouth and never knowing if a word will come out—and if it does, whether it will be the one intended—only adds to the sense of fear. Embarrassment and humiliation are common emotional responses for those who do not have a "progressive neurodegenerative disease" like Alzheimer's.

Creating a world that is safe and secure is paramount for anyone with a dementia. In this environment, it is important for the person to be reminded that he or she is safe. It is very easy for the person to become overwhelmed by too many stimuli. Keeping sounds in the room to a minimum is critical, for example. What may seem innocuous to others can send the person with dementia into a state of overwhelming anxiety. As a dear friend of mine once told me, "not having anything happening can be a good thing." For persons with a dementia process, a structured environment that is safe and secure and filled with supportive people and things that nourish the soul as well as the body are the ideal. Quiet, peaceful silence can be a powerful tool in the world of dementia.

COMPUTERS

For persons with traumatic brain injuries, strokes, or other disorders which interrupt the communication process, the use of a computer may provide a needed outlet. While this may sound simple to many, it may not to the person who is searching for a way to speak to the outside world. In some instances, it can be the single most important tool for the recovery process in persons with speech problems arising from a traumatic brain injury—especially Shaken Brain Syndrome or a stroke that impairs speech or some other cognitive processes.

ANIMALS, AROMAS, AND CHILDREN

On some level, animals, aromas, and children seem to go together when it comes to accessing the inner world of dementia. [91, 92, 93, 94, 95] Animals have long been known to have a "sixth sense" about what is happening with humans. They respond to a simple touch from the human hand. They are loyal friends. When it comes to getting involved with persons with a dementia process, they provide a calming effect. No words are needed. There is an unseen connection between the two. Recently, efforts were initiated to see if dogs could serve as "dementia companions" much like seeing-eye dogs do for the blind. The jury is still out on this idea, but hopefully it will be found to be effective, because many people suffering with dementia could benefit from this resource—especially those with a dementia process who live alone!

Aromas come from many sources. Think about the smell of that favorite perfume your love was wearing on a very important summer's night; that fresh apple pie coming out of your mother's oven; the fresh air after a spring rain; the aroma of cherry tobacco coming from your grandfather's pipe; the odor coming from the barn where the horses have been; the smell of that wet dog coming in out of the rain; the fragrance of a flower oil; the smell of a child's freshly bathed body. These are just a sample of the aromas—the smells—that can stimulate memories of past events in a person's life. Some may be pleasant while others may not, but each will stimulate areas of the brain that trigger other responses. It is for this very reason that aroma therapies are becoming a newer form of treatment for those with a dementia process.

The smiling face of a small child can bring joy to an elder with a progressive dementia. In countries around the world, the pairing of elders and children has proven to create positive events for both.[96] For example, an elderly grandmother in India whose dementia process led her to become more and more confused and unable to live alone was taken in by one of her three sons who had small children. While the other two sons refused to take their mother into their home, claiming they had small children, the one son who did step up to the task reaped unimaginable rewards for himself and his family. This man witnessed his two-year-old son showing no fear of his confused grandmother. The young boy's eight-year-old sister uncovered a unique way of "communicating" with her demented elder: She began to perform the religious chants that had been a part of her grandmother's life, and when she did, she could see joy in the old woman's face. Soon the two were sharing the chanting ritual each day. The younger one would begin the chants and the elder would soon follow. Together they were "communicating" with each other.

In a Kyoto, Japan, group home where elders with dementia reside, young caregivers are taught and encouraged to embrace their charges. The responses are generally big smiles on the faces of those being embraced. Even though such gestures are not customary in the Japanese culture, embraces or hugs are viewed as a form of "non-verbal communication" that allows the younger caregivers and visiting family members opportunities to establish a form of physical contact with the person—a touch—to make a connection with that person who still resides inside the body.[97]

The Hong Kong Alzheimer's Association, in collaboration with local school parent-teacher associations and the Salvation Army, has developed a training program for school children. This program first conducted in Tai Po helps the children to recognize the signs of dementia. With a return response of 92 percent of the surveys on dementia given to the children who participated in this project, eighty-one people in their community received evaluations for cognitive issues. With such a successful outcome, plans are now underway to expand the program across the country. Utilizing children to help identify and locate elders with cognitive decline is a brilliant way to provide early intervention procedures at the local level where many would fall through the cracks. With an increasing number of elderly men and women living alone, programs like this one are going to be needed.[98]

HUMOR

Dr. "Patch" Adams taught the world that children in hospitals can reap physical and psychological benefits from being exposed to humor. He showed everyone that laughter is good medicine! Since then, humor therapy has been incorporated into many different hospital settings.

This same idea has found its way into centers that care for individuals with dementia. In Canada, doctors from the University of Windsor discovered that "clown-doctors" created a positive atmosphere on the units where dementia patients reside. Their tools were simple: smiles and laughter. Studies of their work demonstrated that dementia patients exposed to this "humor therapy" showed improvements in their communications, their recognition of family members, and their memory processes.[99, 100]

Similar results were uncovered in Australia. Dr. Lee-Fay Low from the University of New South Wales School of Psychiatry conduced the SMILE Study across thirty-six Australian residential aged care facilities involved in the recruitment and training of a staff member to act as a "Laughter Boss."[101, 102] This Laughter Boss worked with a humor practitioner with comedic and improvisational skills to provide a playful relationship with residents and staff with a special focus on the residents with dementia.

Those involved in the care of persons with dementia are well aware of the problems that arise with the onset of an episode of agitation. In fact, nearly 70 to 80 percent of people suffering from dementia will experience bouts of agitation at different times during the course of their disease process. Agitated behaviors seen in this group include physical and verbal aggression, wandering, screaming, and repetitive behaviors, just to name a few. Historically, these behaviors are managed with antipsychotic medications which come with the potential for serious side effects.

In Dr. Low's research into the benefits of humor therapy and a Laughter Boss, her study found a 20-percent reduction in agitation when humor therapy was used. This finding was an improvement that was comparable to the use of anti-psychotic medications. The study also showed that agitation in patients with dementia decreased during the twelve-week humor therapy research program and remained lower at the twenty-six-week follow-up evaluation. Happiness and positive behaviors rose on the units over the twelve weeks of the program but dropped soon after the humor therapist's visits stopped.

FLASH CARDS

For many, the repeated asking of the same question over and over again by an Alzheimer's patient can drive a caregiver to near distraction! While many try to answer the question again and again in hopes that something will "register" and the repetitive cycle of the same question will stop, it never works.

A lovely caregiver came up with a simple and novel way to address this problem. She created a series of "Flash Cards" with simple answers to the commonly asked questions that many Alzheimer's patients ask. Each time a person begins to ask the same question over and over, a flash card with the answer is given to the person. It appears to help end the repetitive questioning process. The person with the dementia can look at the card and "know where they are going" or "know the answer to where is Sadie, my wife." For those who cannot afford to purchase a set of these flash cards from the Alzheimer's Association, simple 5x7 index cards will accomplish the same goal.

GRIEVE THE LOSSES AND CELEBRATE THE ASSETS

Loss is *always* a part of any dementia process! Reality changes! What life was like *before* the dementia process becomes history. For those with a disease that creates a progressive degenerative neurological type of dementia process, life moves in a downward spiral. For those with a dementia process that is created by trauma, the course is different. Some of their intellectual and behavioral abilities may eventually return. The same questions come up for both groups. Will anything ever be the same? How long will this go on? Why are some days better than others? These questions all speak to losses that come with a dementia process, regardless of its origin. Metaphorically, these losses are part of a "death process" in the relationships and lives of all who are affected long before the end actually comes. At some point, grieving these losses becomes an important part of a healing process! Holding on to "what was" only prolongs the grieving process.

People with a dementia process most often *live in the here and now*. For those who can recall what life was like before a brain injury, there is a sadness that comes with recognizing the changes. At the same time, they are trying to cope with the challenge of getting from point A to point B or remembering what to do next. For those with a progressive dementia process, more often than not, they do not realize there was a past. For this group there is *only the here and now*. There is no past. There is no tomorrow. In some ways that is a blessing for them. For their loved ones, it usually brings a sadness that creeps into every day.

With these losses come the grief reactions that Dr. Kübler-Ross identified so many years ago: shock, denial, anger, bargaining, and resolution. People get stuck in their grief processes if they are not allowed the opportunity to deal with them. The etiology of the dementia process will dictate the type of grief processes that appear.

Family members of those with a progressive neurodegenerative dementia such as Alzheimer's experience many different levels of grief reactions. I can still recall the woman whose husband was in our Alzheimer's Clinic for a follow-up evaluation of the progression of his disease. They had been married for sixty years. His Alzheimer's had been diagnosed nine years earlier. During this time she had watched the only man she had ever loved in her seventy-six years of life slip away. She knew intimately about the "Long Goodbye"! During our conversation she talked about her deeply held religious beliefs and her frustrations with her husband's disease. Finally, with tears streaming down her face, she blurted out, "I wish that he would go on and die. The man I married is gone. I am embarrassed to say that. It is not the Christian thing to say out loud, but that is the way I feel inside." She sobbed for quite a while. When the time came for her to rejoin her husband, she turned and thanked me for listening to her say things that she couldn't say to other people. For a brief moment in her life, she was allowed to "grieve the loss of her husband."

Little did this devoted wife and grief-stricken woman realize the impact she had on others—especially me! It was that encounter that led me to write my first book about the spiritual aspects of Alzheimer's disease! It also helped to shape the material covered in this book. Her words are still with me—twenty years later!

Celebrating the assets may sound like an odd thing to say when it comes to a dementia process, regardless of its origin. Yet it is an important part of life and living, even with dementia. Every person has assets! Those assets are what each of us is left with at the end of the day. For those of us with the cognitive processes that remain after traumatic brain injury, there are pieces of life to accentuate. We learn to work with what cognitive skills we have remaining and adapt to those that were lost. When I think about this aspect of dementia, I am always reminded of those elders who came before me. They always said, "Dance if you can still dance. Write if you can still write. Play if you can still play. Swim if you still can. Walk if you can. Smile if you can. Breathe each day if that is all you have the energy to do. There will be joy in whatever you can accomplish in a given day. Celebrate it!" Each day I try to do at least one of those!

Celebrations for anyone with a progressive dementia process will be different over time. Every day the person is alive and with us is a day to celebrate his or her presence! It is an opportunity to create memories of times together. Yes, folks, I am completely aware of those days when there is *nothing to celebrate!* On those days, take a moment at the end of the day to be glad that it is over. Tomorrow is always a new day!

For family members whose loved one has that progressive neurodegenerative dementia disease, like Alzheimer's, the day may bring an opportunity to "take care of unfinished business." Remember that *the person with this type of progressive dementia will not remember a single word after it has been said!* Addressing old hurt feelings that have been festering under the surface for years and getting them spoken aloud can transform a relationship. I have witnessed it many times. As I mentioned earlier, others have reported this same phenomenon to me. The final weeks and hours together can become enjoyable. For others this may not be the case. For them it may simply be the understanding that everything that needed to be said was said, everything that could be done was done, and there is a sense of completion that comes in the end.

SEX

Sexuality is a vital part of life—regardless of age. It is as aspect of human development that is often ignored at various stages of life, especially in late life. In many settings it is still a taboo topic. While it is not within the scope of this section to discuss the nuances of sexuality in adults with a dementia process, it is important to stress that it is still a vital aspect of life for many of these people and their partners. Sexuality and intimacy in dementia patients and their partners needs to be addressed and nurtured.[103, 104, 105, 106, 107, 108] Physiological changes in sexual responses occur normally with the aging process, and the addition of a neurological condition that produces a dementia process will only add more layers to the adjustments that will be required for two people who want to continue sharing that part of their relationship. Modifications of activities, behaviors, and expectations about the sexual aspects of the relationship need to be discussed openly with health-care professionals who are in a position to offer individuals and couples help when possible.

♪

Keep in mind that there are more ways to connect to the inner world of a person with dementia beyond the different ones covered in this section. Music is clearly one of the most powerful - for those who have grown up around it. For others it will be something that taps the person's soul and stimulates memories of earlier days. It will often be associated with the person's passions in life. Those strings that connect to the soul can take any form. Searching for those strings can bring joy to anyone who is willing to search for them.

FIVE

Threads of Dementia Prevention

Love and compassion are necessities, not luxuries.
without them, humanity cannot survive.

—The Dalai Lama

Love and compassion come in many forms. They drive the actions of individuals to do things that might otherwise be ignored. They motivate some to do the research required to eradicate all forms of dementia. They are the driving forces for many caregivers. They are the two most important forces behind any efforts people take to prevent or delay the onset of a dementia such as Alzheimer's. These areas are the focus of this chapter. Even as we go to press, pieces of new information are becoming available to anyone who is willing to seek them out.

With that said, I must stress that *there is no magic pill to prevent Alzheimer's or any other disorder that creates a dementia process.* Likewise, there is *no magic cure for any of the disorders* that create a dementia process. What is available to everyone is a litany of recommendations for lifestyle changes and foods that can have an impact on many of the dementia processes presented earlier. In those cases where the problems arise from a traumatic brain injury or a medical procedure, there is hope for new treatment measures to help alleviate some of the cognitive problems.

What is happening in the world of dementia varies by the disorder. Within the arena of Alzheimer's disease, there is a great deal of activity. Increased media coverage of this disease is producing a greater awareness of its prevalence in our global society. Efforts to identify a simple Alzheimer's blood test are underway at the Texas Alzheimer's Research and Care Consortium, which is working together with the US Alzheimer's Disease Neuroimaging Initiative to come up with the most efficacious blood test that is reliable and valid. It is hoped that such a test is somewhere on the horizon.[109, 110]

In the meantime, a new questionnaire designed to help with the early detection of Alzheimer's disease has been developed.[111] A copy of this questionnaire can be obtained from the source referenced here. (If you take this questionnaire, please discuss your responses with your physician.) In addition, the US Food and Drug Administration has recently approved the use of Amyvid, an F18 radioactive diagnostic agent for imaging Alzheimer's.[112] While it is a new diagnostic tool for the more accurate diagnosis of Alzheimer's disease, it will require the training of medical personnel before they are allowed to utilize it in their medical setting.

As one can quickly see, the current efforts seem to be focused on early detection of Alzheimer's disease. One new story on a possible "cure" for the Alzheimer's created a great deal of excitement when it was announced in early 2012.[113] Researchers are looking into the possible use of an FDA-approved cancer drug called Bexarotene and its ability to rapidly remove beta-amyloid from the brains of animal models with Alzheimer's. At this point in history, it will require a series of human trials to examine the viability for this drug's use with Alzheimer's patients. In short, it will take several years to examine the effects of this drug on humans with Alzheimer's disease. For now the medications that are available for the treatment of Alzheimer's disease symptoms are limited to slowing down the progression of the disease.

For those at risk for a stroke, early detection and treatment of symptoms—such as high blood pressure, high blood sugar levels, high cholesterol levels, obesity, an underlying heart condition, or depression—as well as lifestyle changes are the best methods for curtailing the onset of vascular dementia. As many people know, there is a drug known as TPA which—if given within the first three hours of the onset of a stroke—will minimize the stroke's damaging effects. The key to getting this treatment is early recognition followed by immediate action. According to Dr. Hooman Kemel, a neurologist at the New York–Presbyterian Hospital/ Weill Cornell, the common warning signs of an impending stroke include (1) a sudden onset of numbness or weakness in the face, arm, or leg, especially on one side; (2) sudden confusion or trouble speaking or understanding others; (3) sudden trouble seeing in one or both eyes; (4) sudden trouble walking, dizziness, loss of balance, or coordination, or (5) sudden severe headache with no known cause. "Call for an ambulance to take you for treatment" is the finding of a study Dr. Kemel and his colleagues conducted on stroke patients.[114] A delay can lead to permanent irreversible damage. Need I say more?

With the introduction of antiretroviral medications, those with HIV have been able to live long, productive lives,[115] and the prevalence of AIDS-related dementia has been greatly reduced. Within this arena, there is further news of prevention strategies that have been recently identified. The Fred Hutchinson Center's Statistical Center for HIV/AIDS Research and Prevention reported that a large study by the HIV Prevention Trials Network in 2011 made a major scientific breakthrough. The results of this study indicated that the early use of antiretroviral drugs reduced the heterosexual HIV transmission to uninfected sexual partners by 96 percent. This study involved more than 1,700 couples from nine countries on four continents. According to the researchers who participated in this research project, the study's results have galvanized efforts to end the world's AIDs epidemic in a way that would have been inconceivable even one year ago.[116]

"Chemobrain" has just "recently" been identified by medical professionals as a manifestation of the chemotherapy drugs used to fight cancer. While it has been discussed by patients around the world for many years, it has only recently been given any credence by the medical community. In early 2012, doctors at the prestigious Johns Hopkins Medical Center noted that it is an important issue for cancer patients.[117] The cognitive problems and memory issues these patients experience have a negative impact on the person's quality of life post treatment. More specifically many of these people are left with issues such as problems with concentration, forgetfulness, confusion, and disorientation—after they have battled the cancer that required the treatments. For many, these cognitive problems are unexpected as well as unsettling.

Specialists at the Johns Hopkins Medical Center acknowledge they do not understand what causes these cognitive changes. They are working with other medical researchers to try to uncover the origins of these problems. Until a cause and specific treatment are discovered, post-chemotherapy patients are advised to stick to a daily routine, and use written schedules and written reminders to

Five: Threads of Dementia Prevention

track appointments, important events, and important dates. Post-it notes placed in heavily trafficked areas and erasable boards to jot down information are helpful.

For post-operative open heart patients who experience similar cognitive and memory issues, the news resembles that of persons with Chemobrain. The origins of their cognitive problems are not understood,[118] and no treatments are available. Until there is sufficient cause for further investigation into this area, little will be done. Saving lives with open heart procedures supersede concerns for any cognitive fallout that may follow. In time, this may change as the increased focus on dementia processes becomes more prevalent.

For those with traumatic brain injuries, the outlook is slowly getting better. Thanks to the efforts of the National Football League to put images of Cognitive Traumatic Encepalopathy (CTE) in the media, CTE is creeping into the public's awareness.[119] Increasingly, mainstream television programs are presenting episodes that include former professional football players with evidence of cognitive deterioration arising from CTE and the sad outcomes that follow. Making people aware of the problem is the first step. Once there is momentum built up, steps can be made to create equipment to better protect these gladiators of the twenty-first century. Already, research has been initiated that demonstrates the long-term brain damage that can occur in teens and young children who are playing football in the lower grades. [120, 121, 122, 123]

With the increased numbers of Iraq and Afghanistan war veterans returning home with evidence of Shaken Brain Syndrome, a light has been shone on the growing problems that arise from this form of brain trauma.[124, 125] Not only is the fallout from this condition creating problems for the veterans and their families, it is contributing to the growing numbers of suicides among this population. Shame surrounding the cognitive problems that are created by the brain trauma only adds to the level of depression many veterans experience. *If only these brave veterans could understand that the brain trauma creates the cognitive problems. If only they could realize that some of these problems are temporary and will pass with time. If only they could tell themselves and others that they are not mentally ill—they are coping with the fallout from a brain injury!* Sadly, in our culture the stigma of "mental problems" remains, especially in the military, where it can bring about the end of a soldier's career. For soldiers or veterans with a traumatic brain injury, so much is tied to a speedy recovery. Having to cope with a recovery process that can take months to years is a challenge for them as well as for their family members.

Even today, nearly twenty years after my own encounter with a "shaken brain event," there are still aspects of my own brain dysfunction that cause me embarrassment. Like everyone else, I cope with it. Sometimes I laugh about it. Other times I watch family and friends laugh at my failing ability to remember the simplest things. When my speech is off and the words come out garbled, I make some type of comical gesture to misdirect people! Usually it works: People laugh. I get my message out—or blow off the conversation completely and quit talking all together. Still, inside it hurts to know that my life is not the way it was before. But I am what I am, and life goes on!

The only true prevention efforts available to people who want to ward off a dementia process are lifestyle changes. Rather than reinventing the wheel when it comes to providing you with the scientific evidence to support the types of lifestyle changes you need

Five: Threads of Dementia Prevention

to make, I direct you to an international bestselling book, *100 Simple Things You Can Do to Prevent Alzheimer's and Age-Related Memory Loss* by Jean Carper.[126] In it, she has done an excellent job of covering the current trends in lifestyle changes that help to slow down and/or prevent memory loss. For those who are unable to get their hands on this book, I will cover some of the more common things that are recommended in this book and by medical experts in their respective fields of aging:

1. *Learn to deal with stress.*

    Persistent stress reactions to even the simplest events, like a traffic jam, can be dangerous. They trigger a release of corticosteroids. Over time, chronic stress reactions can destroy brain cells and suppress the growth of new ones, increasing your vulnerability to memory decline and dementia. Seek professional advice if you deal with chronic stress.

2. *Learn to meditate.*

    More and more research is demonstrating that the use of meditation or a form of quiet reflection can lower stress and improve one's overall health.

3. *Check your ankles.*

    Low blood flow in your feet and swelling in your ankles is a clue to trouble in your brain. The theory is that blood vessel health is similar throughout the human body. The degree of clogged arteries and blood flow to the feet can suggest atherosclerotic changes in the cerebral blood vessels. Seek professional advice, increase your exercise, and reduce the amount of salt in your diet.

4. *Eat foods that are filled with antioxidants.*
   Foods such as blueberries, blackberries, raisins, and certain vegetables are filled with antioxidants that can slow down memory decline and help prevent Alzheimer's.

5. *Say yes to chocolate.*
   Cocoa, the main ingredient in chocolate, is filled with high concentrations of antioxidants called flavonoids, which contain powerful heart and brain protective properties.

6. *Get treatment for depression.*
   Depression in older adults is also known as pseudo dementia. It can appear to mimic the signs and symptoms of early Alzheimer's. When treated, the depression goes away as do the signs of a dementia process, and the person can resume a normal life.

7. *Get more education.*
   As we age, our brains shrink. It takes longer to learn new things. Scientists now think that people who engage in active learning can increase their brain size. Learning new things can be as simple as taking dance lessons, taking up a new hobby, doing an Internet search, learning a new game, or taking a class at the local college. Stimulating the brain to learn something new is the key.

8. *Say yes to coffee.*
   Coffee is an anti-inflammatory! It is now viewed as a tonic for the aging brain. It helps to block the effects of

cholesterol in the brain and reduces the risks of stroke, depression, and diabetes.

9. *Know your estrogen levels.*
Since women make up at least sixty to seventy percent of those with Alzheimer's, it is important to know what their estrogen levels are. Why? As women age, they lose the protection of the hormone estrogen which boosts memory. Although the use of estrogen replacement therapy in post-menopausal women is controversial in America, it is a topic that should be discussed with a medical professional.

10. *Follow a Mediterranean diet.*
The food on this diet has consistently been found to help save the brain from memory decline and dementia. The diet is rich is green leafy vegetables, fish, fruits, nuts, legumes, olive oil, and a little wine. Eating these foods can cut the risk of developing Alzheimer's by half.

11. *Get a good night's sleep.*
A good night's sleep has the power to protect the brain against memory loss and Alzheimer's by manipulating the brain's levels of beta-amyloid, the toxic peptide that is a prime factor in Alzheimer's. Research has also found that sleeping an average of five hours or fewer has been linked to large increases in visceral abdominal fat, which can contribute to the development of diabetes and obesity. If you suffer from symptoms of sleep apnea, seek

treatment. It cannot only save your brain, it can reduce stress to your heart and help to prevent heart attacks.

12. *Have a big social circle.*
Although experts in aging, Alzheimer's, and dementia do not yet understand the mystery surrounding it, they do acknowledge that being actively involved in a social circle is "neuro-protective." It creates a strong "cognitive reserve" in those people who consistently and frequently engage in interactions with friends and family members. Experts say that expanding one's social network over time is a key factor is staying alert and warding off Alzheimer's disease. Do not isolate yourself: It can be hazardous to your health.

13. *Take care of your teeth.*
Flossing teeth daily is a key strategy for maintaining a healthy aging body. A little known fact is that the health of the teeth and gums is related to the health of the heart. Dental researchers have found that infections in the gums release inflammatory byproducts that travel to the areas in the brain involved with memory loss. The simple tasks of brushing and flossing daily can help keep your brain healthy and your mental faculties sharper.

14. *Get enough Vitamin B-12.*
Blood levels of Vitamin B-12 go down as we age. According to researchers at Oxford University, brains that operate on low levels of Vitamin B-12 actually shrink. This shrinkage

can lead to brain atrophy by ripping away the myelin, a protective sheath around the neurons. Seek professional advice to get tested for a Vitamin B-12 deficiency and appropriate treatment recommendations.

15. *Put vinegar on/in everything.*

Vinegar cuts risk factors that may lead to memory decline: high blood sugar levels, insulin resistance, diabetes, and weight gain. How? It has a potent glucose-lowering effect and it can curb appetite and food intake. Consequently, it helps to prevent weight gain and obesity, which are associated with diabetes, accelerated dementia, and memory loss. Any type of vinegar works. Use it on foods. Drink a spoonful of it in a glass of drinking water. Just use it!

16. *Eat curry.*

Curry powder contains the spice turmeric, packed with curcumin, a compound reported to stall or delay memory decline. Curcumin appears to work both by blocking the buildup of the Alzheimer's-producing amyloid plaques and by eating away at the existing plaques, thereby slowing cognitive decline.

17. *Drink wine—especially red wine.*

A daily glass of wine may help to delay dementia. Research shows that alcohol—in moderation—is an anti-inflammatory and raises good cholesterol, which helps to ward off dementia. The high antioxidants in red wine give it an added anti-dementia benefit.

18. Drink tea—especially green tea.

Both black and green teas contain compounds that can pass through the blood-brain barrier and block nerve damage. The green tea has the added benefit of an antioxidant that can block the toxicity of beta-amyloid, which kills brain cells. The more tea you drink—black or green—the sharper your aging memory is!

19. Prevent and control diabetes.

Having type 2 diabetes makes you vulnerable to Alzheimer's disease as well as a host of other medical complications. The earlier the diagnosis, the greater the risk, and the higher the odds of getting dementia become. Researchers note that diabetes and Alzheimer's disease have similar causative factors: obesity, high blood pressure, high cholesterol, high-fat and high-sugar diets, low activity levels, and high blood sugar levels. Every effort should be made to prevent the onset of type 2 diabetes. Keep blood sugar levels low; prevent or treat obesity, exercise, and eat foods that help to lower cholesterol levels.

20. Exercise daily.

The benefits of daily exercise and its contribution to the prevention of a dementia process are too numerous to cover in such a short space. All types of exercise are beneficial. A simple fifteen-minute walk each day has been found to provide many beneficial effects in aging adults. It increases heart rate and breathing. It can help curtail weight gain. It can provide a social activity for those who walk in groups. It can be done anywhere. It does not require special equipment. It DOES require that you DO IT. If that is not enough to get you out there walking, listen to this: Not only does exercise increase endorphin levels in the brain that make you feel good, it stimulates a hormone in the blood that helps with the long-term recovery from a stroke. Experts in all areas of aging agree that *exercise is the simple most important activity to improve and maintain a healthy body* as we all age across the decades.

21. *Recognize memory problems.*

Early detection of problems with memory can be important. *For those with a true Alzheimer's disease process, the lack of recognition of any memory problems is a cardinal sign.* For those with an undiagnosed depression, treatment of the underlying problem can eliminate the memory problems. If you are concerned that you may have a medical problem that can produce a dementia process, seek out a medical professional who knows how to diagnose dementia. For those with memory problems related to a traumatic brain injury, seek out professionals who can help to accurately identify the specific problems you are having. Ask for recommendations for appropriate treatments. Be aware that you may have to search out treatments on your own.

The same holds true for those with memory problems related to chemotherapies and/or open heart procedures.

Other recommendations for preventing dementia come from a variety of other sources:

1. *Pay attention to your vision and hearing care.*
   Some recent research out of Canada suggests that aging adults who take care of the vision and hearing, to include proper fitting dentures and hearing aids, appear to lower their risk of developing dementia at a later point. The researchers looked at very large sample of people free of dementia over a ten year period. While they acknowledge that more research needs to be done in this area, it stands to reason that taking care of all aspects of one's health over time can help to prevent problems ahead of time.[127]

2. *Use everyday memory boosters.*
   Dr. Peter Rabins and his team at the Johns Hopkins School of Medicine offer a series of simple techniques to help all aging adults improve their memory and maintain a handle on their day-to-day lives.[128] Staying focused, active, and alert are the three key factors to remember. Beyond these, they recommend the following techniques:
   - Place commonly lost items in a designated place
   - Write things down
   - Say words out loud
   - Use memory aids—e.g., cell phones, notepads, wrist watch alarms, calendars for appointments
   - Use visual aids
   - Group items using mnemonics (procedures or words that help trigger the memory)
   - Concentrate and relax
   - Get plenty of sleep

Five: Threads of Dementia Prevention

3. *Feed your brain.*

The brain needs protein to build cells, to produce chemicals necessary for nerves to communicate, and to repair damage. The sources for this protein are under some measure of scrutiny at this point. Some diets that are recommended for other known medical conditions—e.g., heart disease—may deprive the brain of proteins and the related fats needed for their proper function. It is not my place to recommend one diet over another. What is important here is that you look further into the types of foods that your body requires to treat the physical disorders/conditions you have. Seek a medical professional for any questions and recommendations you might have. It may help you to know that medical professionals are learning more and more about the effects of nutritional habits and the healing contributions different food groups can make to our bodies.

At this juncture, some of you might expect me to discuss the different types of complementary supplements, such as gingko balboa, and their contributions to memory health. Research on these compounds is still underway by reputable medical institutions. Because many of them may be contraindicated when used with many prescription medications, I can only recommend that you speak with your personal physician about these. With their increasing use—by many adults of all ages—medical professionals are finally beginning to collect information about their patients' supplement use before they initiate any medical treatment plan. Working together is definitely the way to get the best medical care for any individual.

Prevention measures for all conditions that produce dementia processes are ongoing. Those who are susceptible to events that can produce a traumatic brain injury need to be aware of ongoing research efforts at major medical centers across America. These specialists are trying to identify strategies that can prevent brain shearing that can occur inside of the skull while the head is still inside of the helmet of anyone who undergoes a shaken brain event. Until they are successful, every effort to prevent a head trauma must be taken.

SIX

Caregivers: Our Unsung Heroes

Those who have done the impossible
often didn't know it was impossible when they did it!

—The Prophet of Life

During the weeks and months that followed the 9/11 attack in New York City, many tributes to those who died and those who helped with the recovery process were shown on television. It was a hard time for all of us. One tribute for the many dogs on the K-9 teams who helped locate the missing people in the Twin Towers rubble struck me as very poignant. As a nation we were honoring all who had helped that day and the many days that followed, even the smallest of them all—the dogs!

As I watched those beautifully prepared television pieces, I was grateful for the honors bestowed upon those courageous animals. They had truly performed miracles during that very difficult period. It got me to thinking about other heroes in our everyday lives whom no one ever recognizes. I had just signed a contract to write a book on a topic that was dear to my heart, Caregiver Compassion Fatigue©. All of the "appropriate research" had been done. I was ready to write about how caregivers were undergoing a form of fatigue that was not being recognized by anyone. As they give their all to the person(s) in their care—in this case, persons with Alzheimer's—they eventually find themselves worn out and in great despair. For Alzheimer's care, it is a one-way street for the caregiver. At some point, there is nothing left to give. Still there are expectations that remain. "I must continue on—somehow" is a common theme I have heard over the years. "Continuing on" may last for years!

What I repeatedly heard caregivers telling me was "I give and I give (to this person with dementia) until I have nothing left. I love him/her but that is not enough. It's this process of constantly giving and never getting anything back in return that is taking its toll on me. There is no relief in sight. I don't know how I will make it, but I will find a way." This is what I have labeled as Caregiver Compassion Fatigue.© It is not a "burnout process," like so many people try to label it. It is a condition of "imbalance that comes from the unending process of constantly giving every day" that is profoundly unique to caregivers—especially those caring for a person with dementia. It is a form of unending stress! Not surprisingly, many caregivers are developing their own dementia process as a "reward" for their selfless giving.

As I prepared to write my book manuscript in 2001, I tried out the material on a small group at a nearby church. There were many seniors in the audience who were caring for a spouse at that very moment. When I told them they were heroes, they looked at me with shock and surprise. No one had ever said anything like that to them. How could *they* be *heroes* when they were just doing what came naturally to them. They were taking care of someone they loved.

Six: Caregivers

When I pointed out that they were members of a "worldwide group of people" who were doing the same thing "in silence," they sat up in their seats. Some mumbled, "I didn't know that. I thought it was just me out there doing it." In truth, they were and still are part of a rapidly growing segment of our global society. With each passing year, the numbers swell. The following are just a few of the known facts that I shared with my audience that day. (The numbers have been updated for this publication.)

1. Over 15 million Americans provide unpaid care for a single person with Alzheimer's disease or other dementias. The numbers of these same types of caregivers in other countries are still relatively unknown or are still being collected by their health officials.

2. Unpaid caregivers are primarily a family member, relative, or friend.

3. These caregivers are more likely to be females (fifty-two years and older) and married.

4. They provide an average of 21.9 hours of direct care per week. The hours are greater if the person with dementia lives in the home with the caregiver.

5. This care is valued at $12.12/hour by US experts. That comes to $265.43 USD per week or $13,802.36 USD per year in unpaid care that is given to each person with Alzheimer's disease or another form of dementia. Be aware that some people can live with Alzheimer's disease for up to twenty years![129]

As my audience members heard these simple facts roll off my tongue, their faces took on a new demeanor. There was pride in their eyes. As they took in this information, they began to realize a truth. *They are heroes!* They do something extraordinary that very few people notice. They give freely of themselves to another person. They do not expect anything in return. They do what is required of them with what they have. In most cases, they do it all out of love.

On that day, I knew that I had struck a chord. I was excited. Only days later as I was making preparations to stop everything and write my wonderful book of wisdom, an event happened that would teach me new lessons about caregiving and Caregiver Compassion Fatigue© that were not in the research books or magazines I had read.

Michael, my husband, fell gravely ill after a minor outpatient surgical procedure. He was diagnosed with Myeolodysplasia, a form of bone marrow cancer. (Yes, this is the same disease Robin Roberts of ABC's *Good Morning America* is battling.) I became my husband's sole caregiver for the next nine months. When he wasn't in hospitals receiving treatments for a progressively failing health process, we were traveling around the USA exploring treatment options for him.

In no time, I was carrying around a canvas bag filled with weekly medical reports and treatment recommendations. After it grew to four inches in width, I had to get another bag to hold the new medical documents that were added. With all of the changes occurring in American health care, I quickly learned to become a "health care patient advocate" before there was such an animal. I carried lists of doctors who had treated Michael. I carried lists of medications that had been tried and discarded. I carried lab reports from every hospital that had done a bone marrow aspiration or drawn blood for this test or that. There were also insurance forms. There were multiple copies

Six: Caregivers

of personal identification for this registration desk or that one. It was a never-ending nightmare for both of us. Finally, I dropped everything I was trying to do and became a full-time caregiver, nurse, patient advocate, and administrative assistant.

Over the course of these events, I tried many of the "wonderful pieces of wisdom for caregivers" that I was planning to put into my new book. It was all CRAP! None of it worked! There was no time for taking walks in the park. There was no place to sit quietly and deep breathe for a few minutes. I was "on" 24/7! No one came to relieve me.

Both of our families lived far away. None of them had the financial resources to come and help me with Michael's care. Does this sound familiar to any of you who are caring for a loved one with a dementia process or any other failing health problem?

There were medications to deliver. IV's had to be changed. Nutritious foods had to be delivered in a palatable form. I was not the best cook, so that was always a challenge. It was during this period that I learned about the healing powers of blueberries, blackberries, and other fruits. For Michael, there was no definitive cure for his illness short of a bone marrow transplant—which he received later that year.

Eventually, I learned that the universe seems to have a way of providing us with what we need and teaching us new things along the way. Seven months into our healthcare quest for a cure, we had to travel to Seattle for the bone marrow transplant. Michael was surrounded by the best of the best medical experts in the world. As a caregiver, like so many of you, I was expected to look after my husband. The focus was always on him. For that I was very grateful. There was not time for me to do anything but give care where I could and support my husband through his treatment.

To my utter amazement, two very special social workers assigned to our case pulled me aside one day at the cancer care clinic. They honored me by telling me what they observed about me during that period. I was stressed. My husband was an unusually intellectually gifted man who was extremely hard to care for. The transplant clinic staff required their own therapy sessions with a psychiatrist to help them deal with him. These two wonderful women told me in no uncertain terms that I could not keep up the pace of care that was going to be needed after the transplant procedure was completed. Somehow they convinced me to "let them take care of my husband" for a few short hours each week.

Just hearing their words gave me a measure of relief that was indescribable. Finally, there was some help "for me."

During that period, it was a lonely journey both for Michael and for me. We only had each other to lean on. That is the way it had always been for us through the years. Everyone at the transplant center was doing their best to keep him alive and get him through the arduous treatment program. I had long since given up any hope of thinking that anyone would notice how my life was operating in a vacuum! Those two women did, though. They were angels to me. They offered some recommendations on things I could do to get some true relief for myself.

Below are some of the techniques they recommended. From one caregiver to another, I hope these offer you some help *and* some relief.

1. *Let someone help you with your caregiving tasks.*

    Get some help, if only for a few hours each week. This will require that you allow someone else to "take charge" and relieve you of your caregiving duties for a while—not replace you.

2. *Get a handicap sticker/card.*
   Ask the physician who is providing health care for you and your loved one to give you a signed authorization form for a handicap sticker/card to place in your automobile. Take it to your local government office that issues the automobile tags for your car. Get a handicap sticker/card, put it into the front windshield of your car, and use the handicap parking spaces where ever you go. Over time you will find that it provides you with some small measure of assistance. You will be closer to the buildings. It makes life easier for you when it comes to getting your loved one in and out of the car to go anywhere, especially for visits to the doctor's office, to the laboratory, to the hospital.

3. *Take yourself out for some "Retail Therapy."*
   Each week I took a shuttle bus into town and walked up and down streets looking at window displays. When I felt like it, I would walk into a store and look at the new clothes, the new shoes, or the new crafts on display. On very rare occasions, I would make a small purchase. Money was tight and I did not have a nickel to waste. Still, the very process of walking down a street, looking at new things, and strolling among unfamiliar people going about their business gave me some relief. My stress level went down.

4. *Eat some chocolate.*
   Each night I would eat four small pieces of Dove chocolate from a bag someone had given me. When that bag ran out, I bought a new one. Why? Inside each wrapper was a short

message of encouragement. I needed encouragement and support from anywhere that I could get it. The Dove Candy Company became one of my support systems! How's that for an odd twist of fate! Soon, I was taking those encouraging messages from the chocolate wrappers with me to the hospital. While Michael was getting his chemotherapy treatments, I was writing a new message on an erasable board in his hospital room each day. Soon the doctors and nurses were coming into Michael's room just to see what new message was on the board. One day, one of the residents pulled me aside and told me the entire medical staff looked forward to reading my little messages. He said that it was a bright spot in their otherwise challenging days on the chemotherapy unit of the hospital.

5. *Go somewhere quiet and have a good cry!*
This approach may be used as often as needed. It provides an emotional release as well as a physical expression of your pent-up stresses. It requires no assistance. A box of Kleenex is recommended. Sometimes those crying episodes can go on for a while. You can then pull yourself together and get back to the business at hand after you have finished.

6. *Eat a nourishing meal every day.*
Ideally, you should get a plate of good food into your body every day. You have to maintain your own health and nourishment throughout the caregiving period—however long it is. Eating out from time to time can also provide you with some relief. In some parts of America as well as some

Six: Caregivers

other countries, dementia cafés are appearing. They provide an outing for both the caregiver as well as the person with dementia. If there is nothing like that near you, allow someone to stay with your loved one while you go out for a meal. If you can have company, the social interactions with another person who is not caught up in the world of dementia can be a welcomed distraction. For me, it was a quiet meal that someone else prepared. I quickly appreciated the experience. To this day, ten years later, I still enjoy a lunch on my own. People watching can be fun, and eating someone else's cooking is always a treat.

7. *Let someone else clean your space.*

    For me, having a housekeeper coming into the hotel room where we lived during the transplant process was such a gift to me. It was one less thing I had to do each day. It was also a relief to return to our room each day and find everything cleaned and in perfect order. Many times during that period, I would recall a conversation I had years earlier with a stately gentleman in Kentucky whose wife had Alzheimer's disease. He wanted to bring in a housekeeper for his wife. She could no longer manage their household. It was one thing that he could still give her. Having a clean and orderly space each day for a person whose life is filled with daily chaos can be the simplest and most profound gift.

8. *Get a good night's sleep.*

    For Alzheimer's caregivers, this may be a near-impossible task but one that must be addressed. Regardless of the situation that you are dealing with, it is imperative that you get sleep. If necessary, seek professional help with strategies for ensuring that both you and your loved one get several hours of sleep each night. Recently, I was made aware of some centers that are offering what they advertise as "day care services" for seniors with dementia—"*at night.* The new service allows caregivers to rest and get a good night of sleep while the loved one with dementia is monitored by another set of caregivers at the center. In the "day care service center" at night, the person with dementia can roam freely about the center, receive a meal, and be returned home in the morning to a caregiver who is rested and ready to take on the new day.

9. *Let some things go.*
The life of a caregiver—regardless of his or her reasons for taking on this role—is no longer the same as it was! Daily routines will change. Some things that were once "necessary" will need to fall by the wayside. Trying to keep up with life "the way it was" will not work! There will be tasks, events, and/or personal and situational demands on your time that will have to be stopped or dropped. You will have to learn to "let them go." In the grand scheme of things, they really won't/don't matter anyway. This is a hard thing to do for many of us.

10. *Give your own body some TLC/special care.*
Your special care will be something that is meaningful and stress-reducing to you. For me, walking was a challenge.

Six: Caregivers

Every day I found myself too exhausted to walk anywhere that I did not have to go. Running was out of the question. Both were pieces of that "recommended wisdom" I was going to write about before! At some point, I found a wonderful young massage therapist from Romania who worked at a small spa in a nearby mall. She gave me the best deep tissue massages every week. She was truly a life safer. For at least two or three hours after my massage, the stress was gone. I felt at peace with the world. My body was relaxed. I could feel my limbs. Food had taste. Eventually, the numbness of my entire body would return as my caregiving duties took center stage again. It was always very easy for me to shut down my mind and my body so that I could focus on the tasks at hand. That was one of my coping methods. On some rare occasions, I found some stress relief by spending time splashing around in the hotel's swimming pool.

While these things worked for me in my situation, they may not be options for you. Take a look at the methods you use to cope with your routine caregiving responsibilities. Take a look at your life, your world, your environment. Find things that work for you to help you relax. Keep them simple; they do not have to cost a lot of money. Here are some examples: Get your hands into the dirt by planting a flower garden. Grow a vegetable garden. Visit with a friend. Bake a pie. Go fishing. Go to a baseball game. Go to see a funny movie. Go to your place of worship and spend some quiet time there. Whatever you choose to do, make sure that it brings *you* relief and joy!

11. *Stay connected to others.*

    This can take any form that you choose. Call someone on the phone The call does not have to be a long one, but just hearing another human's voice often brings a subtle measure of pleasure. Write letters. Send E-mails. Join Facebook or Twitter and send messages via these social media outlets. Let people know how to contact you. If you are not the caregiver and want to provide support to a caregiver you know, send cards from time to time. Send prayers for all involved. They do work in ways that scientists do not yet fully understand. The bottom line is to stay connected to others. The social support is very important!

12. *Manage the family drama.*

    Nearly all of us have it. It can be taxing and draining. Caregiving is hard enough on its own without the emotional drama that arises when a family member develops a life threatening illness that can have a protracted period of decline. Commonly, among persons with Alzheimer's disease, one person becomes the "designated caregiver." Everyone else is too busy, too far away, too *something* to take on the requirements needed to provide the day-to-day care. The dynamics of the family system get turned upside down. Rather than banding together to help each other, a lot of "should have, would have, or could have done this or that" emerges. If you are the caregiver, let these statements go and remain focused on your loved one's needs. Try to adjust your expectations of others. In some instances *you may even need to eliminate any expectations* from your family members. It may be the only coping strategy that you have available to you.

13. *Stay on top of Legal and financial documents.*

In each country the types of documents for overseeing the care of someone with a dementia process will vary according to the laws of that country and municipality. Ask the appropriate sources for guidance. If you are in doubt, contact one of the international organizations listed in the Resources section at the end of this book. In the United States, the following documents will be needed at some point. The sooner they are prepared, the easier it will be for everyone. These documents include a Durable Power of Attorney for Medical Decisions, Durable Power of Attorney for Financial Decisions, a Living Will, and a Final Will and Testament that outlines the distribution of the person's assets at the time of their death. In many states, a document that gives guardianship may be required if the loved one is no longer able to make decisions on his or her own. Be aware that a diagnosis of Alzheimer's disease does not automatically render that person incompetent to make decisions and sign legal documents.

Once each of these documents has been prepared, make copies and put the originals into a safe place. Different health care providers will ask for copies of one or more of these documents over the course of an individual's treatment program.

Financial documents are often maintained by one person in a relationship. If that person develops a dementia process, those duties will fall to someone else. In most cases that will be the spouse, the partner, or an adult child. It is imperative that the other person who assumes these responsibilities be cognizant of the monthly income and expenses as well as the location of any life insurance documents, property deeds, health insurance cards, etc. Organize all of these documents and place them in one location. Keep up with all monthly invoices, bank statements, and other communications that relate to important documents.

Educate yourself to the types of scams that may be going on in your area or over the Internet. Aging adults and those with a dementia process are a growing niche for con men and women who are kind, friendly, and exceedingly skillful at stealing the assets of their victims.

14. *Keep a journal.*

Writing your thoughts in a journal each night may be the only option you have for gaining some emotional relief from your caregiver duties. Some very important research out of Southern Methodist University in Dallas, Texas, has demonstrated the healing effects of writing down one's thoughts and feelings.[130,131,132,133] This simple action delivers a chemical change in the human blood-stream that helps to promote stress relief.

15. *Honor your work. Honor your accomplishments.*
    Accept and honor that you are a true hero.

Each person who serves as a caregiver is a hero! Alzheimer's disease caregivers and those who provide care to a person with a dementia process fall into this special category of Caregiver Heroes. The tasks they deliver each day are only surpassed by the level of challenges they must face. Every person's dementia process is unique. Each has its own set of specific behavioral and emotional disturbances. Each person's care will vary by disease, by setting, by financial resources, by support systems that are—or are not—available, and by the medical care that is—or is not—available. In every case, it is the accomplishment(s) made each day that add up over time. One day it may simply mean the caregiver made it through the day without a major crises popping up out of the blue. Another day, there may be a moment in time where that very demented person shows a single sign of recognition—just a smile, perhaps.

Whatever your caregiving situation requires, know that others do take notice. Pat yourself on the back from time to time. When your caregiving days come to an end, know that you are a hero in that person's eyes.

♪

Caring for a person with dementia is challenging. I don't care what medical condition creates the intellectual and behavioral changes in the individual's dementia process. Each day the demands placed on the caregiver and his or her charge will vary. There will be good days. Joyful things *might* happen. Cherished memories *may* be created. Other days are filled with one stressful challenge after another. These are the rough days. Every caregiver has them. Some caregiving periods will be short – only weeks or months. Others will last for years – even decades. Life and relationships will change. Taking care of a person with dementia routinely falls to the spouse, partner or a single family member who is always viewed as the "caretaker" of the family. It usually goes unnoticed by others. Taking care of the caregiver is not a priority – in anyone's book. Even many caregivers will ignore their own needs.

These unsung heroes need care and attention just like their charges. They need to "take care of themselves" too. The different methods I listed in this section worked for me. They are simple and easy to do. They made a difference in my caregiving situation - which only lasted a year. Others will need different forms of care because theirs will be longer. Their settings will be different. They may not have the resources of a large city and an urban hospital setting like I did. Many live in places where they must draw on their surroundings for support and relief. Regardless of the setting, caregivers need some form of support, attention and relief and relaxation to recharge their own souls from time to time.

At some point, every person's caregiving demands come to an end. All that remains are memories of the person they knew – with and without the dementia. Oddly, in these situations our minds have a way of letting only the good times be remembered. They are the ones that seem to be cherished. They are the ones that make us smile in the quiet moments.

SIX: CAREGIVERS

"Moments Like These (Will Never End)"
Excerpt of lyrics by Alan DeValle

> Come and let us wander.
> Let's walk inside the footsteps of the day.
> Take the time to wonder, too…
> Go barefoot like a child gone out to play.
>
> Time goes racing by,
> I don't know why
> We let it slip away.
> Come and share the treasures
> We can find in every day.
>
> Moments like these will never end.
> Come feel the breeze,
> It's whispering, "I love you."
> Look at the stars!
> Each one is your friend.
> Shining so far, so high,
> So bright above you.
>
> May you always know the kiss
> Of a moment such as this…

Permission granted by Diamond in the Rose Publishing

SEVEN

Dementia in the 21st Century

The pursuit of happiness is the chase of a lifetime to become what you "might have been."

—Unknown Author

In the spring of 2012, the World Health Organization announced that dementia is reaching epidemic levels. Dementia therefore needs to become a public health priority. Worldwide, nearly 35.6 million people live with dementia. These numbers are expected to double by 2030 to 65.7 million and triple by 2050 to nearly 115.4 million people. Treating and caring for people with dementia *currently costs* the world nearly US$604 billion dollars each year. (Recall that each US household provides approximately $13,000 per year in *unpaid care!*). Those who are looking at this issue acknowledge that raising public awareness about dementia, early detection of its presence, and strategies to reduce and eliminate the stigma that is associated with it are mandatory.[134]

Increasingly, the elderly are left alone to care for themselves in America as well as in other countries around the world. This fact comes from the growing trends of fewer children being born to each couple, a staggering increase in divorces, fewer three-generational households with the elders living on their own, an increase in the number of women returning to the work force, and more young people migrating to cities and leaving many of their elders isolated in rural settings. These are just a few of the trends that are creating more pressure on caregivers and increasing the likelihood that many elders will simply have no relatives around to care for them.[135] As the numbers of people with a dementia process continue to grow and the healthcare funds in each country continue to dwindle or dry up completely in some areas of the world, spending resources to prolong the lives of feeble elders with dementia will probably receive more scrutiny.

Efforts are underway to improve the health of aging adults in many parts of the world. Better health, improved diets, and lifestyle changes will certainly help reduce the prevalence of dementia in the coming decades. The topics that follow demonstrate some of the simple things that can be done in our communities.

EXERCISE

A new study by researchers at the Vancouver Coastal Health and University of British Columbia in Canada shows how creating a seniors' exercise program that specifically includes the use of resistance training can help to alter the physical decline in this group. Beyond the physical benefits of their resistance training, the participants displayed an improvement in their executive cognitive processes of selective attention, conflict resolution functions, and associative memory.[136]

DIET

Beyond incorporating various types of exercise and increasing one's social network, consuming a variety of different foods seems to be the other "best approach" to staving off memory decline as well as various medical conditions that create a dementia process. The material that follows addresses the findings of some of the latest research in this area.

Berries: Consuming high amounts of blueberries and strawberries can protect against memory decline in women, according to an article published in the April 26, 2012 issue of *Annals of Neurology.* Dr. Elisabeth Devore of Brigham and Women's Hospital and Harvard Medical School examined results from a longitudinal study of nurses that began in 1976. She and her colleagues reviewed the dietary questionnaires that were collected over the years by the study's participants. Cognitive function was tested every two years in 16,010 participants who were seventy years of age between 1995 and 2001. As already stated, they found that the consumption of high amounts of these berries were associated with a significantly slower decline in the cognitive function test scores. In their study are references to additional biological evidence which supports their findings.[137]

Coffee: In a special supplement to the *Journal of Alzheimer's Disease,* "Therapeutic Opportunities for Caffeine in Alzheimer's Disease and Other Neurodegenerative Diseases," several international experts from Portugal and other countries around the world present information on the effects of coffee on the brain. Several key findings of their research include the following:

- There are multiple beneficial effects of caffeine that normalize brain function and prevent its generation.

- A neuroprotective profile for caffeine has been established.
- Epidemiological studies corroborated by meta-analysis suggest that caffeine may be protective against Parkinson's disease.
- Caffeine as a candidate disease-modifying agent for Alzheimer's disease was presented.[138, 139, 140]

Nuts: Research studies on the neuroprotective effects of different types of nuts do exist. Some of the more common nuts reviewed are almonds and pecans. Both have been found to offer beneficial effects on aging adults.[141] It is not within the scope of this section to discuss all of them. If you are interested in these studies, I recommend contacting your local Alzheimer's Association.

Coconut oil: A brilliant physician whose husband had dementia conducted her own single case study on the use of coconut oil as a treatment strategy. Dr. Mary Newport began this research in 2001 after reading an article published by Dr. Richard L. Veech of the National Institutes of Health entitled "Ketone bodies, potential therapeutic uses." Her husband had a progressive dementia for at least five years. She described his life as being one in which many days he was in a fog and could not figure out how to get water out of the refrigerator or even find a spoon. On other days he could remember things and appeared to be his normal happy self. To learn about the many improvements her husband has experienced since she began using coconut oil in his diet, read her well-written book entitled *What If There Was a Cure for Alzheimer's Disease and No One Knew?* You may be quite intrigued by her findings. After two years of a daily dose of coconut oil, she has carefully documented that her husband has improved dramatically, jogs again, reads and remembers what he has read, gets distracted less often, and has had a stable MRI for the entire two-year period.[142]

Since Dr. Newport began talking publicly about the benefits of coconut oil use with dementia, there has been a growing interest in what dementia researchers call the "Keto-Dementia Diet."[143] While the jury is still out on this approach, researchers have reported that the ketogenic diet does appear to have neuroprotective effects. It is an area worth exploring for those who believe that it may offer some benefit.

HORMONES

Dr. Mark L. Gordon, an interventional endocrinologist in Los Angeles, California, sustained a closed head injury several years ago. This event led to his discovery that traumatic brain injuries can alter hormone functioning. After doing extensive research within the medical literature, he identified a condition he calls "Traumatic Brain Injury Hormone Dysfunction Syndrome." Over time he developed a treatment approach that is based on the TBI patient's specific hormonal imbalances.[144] He is currently engaged in a national study that involves the medical testing of war veterans who are suffering from TBI-related injuries as well as non-veterans with traumatic brain injuries who meet the criteria for the study's treatment protocols. To learn more about TBI Hormone Dysfunction Syndrome and Dr. Gordon's research study, see www.tbilegal.com.

GENE THERAPY

Good news continues to pour out of the dementia research community. Researchers in the United States and Europe have discovered a "genetic mutation" they say protects against Alzheimer's disease and holds promise for a possible treatment for this dreaded disease.[145] While this latest finding has just been made public, it offers hope for a future without Alzheimer's in the twenty-first century.

DANCING

The results of a 21-year study of seniors conducted by researchers at the Albert Einstein College of Medicine in New York City found that reading, playing board games, and playing musical instruments were associated with a lower risk of dementia.[146] Of the eleven different physical activities examined in this study, dancing was the *only one* associated with a lower risk of dementia! The other physical activities studied e.g. walking, swimming, playing tennis or golf produced more cardiovascular benefits than cognitive ones. These researchers suggest the reason dancing has such a positive effect is that it frequently creates new neural pathways. How? Dancing is not automatic. Decisions about what dance step comes next must be made within split seconds. This process stimulates the brain!

According to Dr. Peter Davies, an Alzheimer's expert who recently spoke at the twenty-fifth annual meeting of the New York City Alzheimer's Chapter, dancing is clearly the best method we have for dementia prevention.[147] It sounds like putting on your dancing shoes and getting out on the floor can be fun *and* healthy!

♪

While the researchers are hard at work to identify new ways to detect, slow down, and eliminate all of the neurodegenerative diseases and traumatic brain injuries that produce a dementia process, we are charged with taking those steps toward prevention that are within our

Seven: Dementia in the 21st Century

own power. Many of those steps have already been identified in early sections: Educate yourself on dementia. Stay connected with anyone who has a dementia process. Utilize those measures—e.g., exercise, social networks, and appropriate foods—to slow down and improve the cognitive function of every adult. Help to eliminate the stigma associated with dementia because it is going to become a common feature in all of our lives—if it is not already!

EPILOGUE

A year ago when I began writing this book, the goals were simple: Educate readers on dementia! Show them what it looks like, how to prevent it, and how to work with it when it does appear. Above all, try to help eliminate the stigma associated with any dementia process!

Along the way, the writing process took on a life of its own, as all books do. Trying to use a very linear approach to this creative project only frustrated me. Trying to digest the wealth of updated research materials I had collected was nearly impossible. At different points, I had to step away from the materials and the process of writing. I continued to re-examine the approach I was trying to use. What was my message? There was so much information about the diseases that were selected for this book. The linear process of looking at all of this material I had been taught in school was not working.

Eventually, I began to look at the commonalities of each of the different conditions that created dementia. At first it was a mystery. I had to ask myself the following questions: What was the single most common thread that tied them all together? What threads could be plucked from our lives that would allow those on the outside to remain connected to the inner world of those with dementia? All the while as I examined these questions, more and more information became available on the different types of dementias.

Finally, I recognized that writing this book was an organic process. Just as each person's dementia process takes twists and turns, this book was unfolding with material that would require different pathways. As a writer, I had to trust the creative process that was happening and know that I would do the work that was required. Each caregiver does this same thing every day. Hopefully, we both end up with something that we can be proud of when all is said and done.

Within the pages of this book, I have tried to communicate some very simple messages about dementia. How each reader utilizes that information will be different. One's life experiences will help shape how each person makes sense of the information presented on each page. For some, the messages will be crystal clear. For others, parts will be confusing in some places—especially the discussions about spirit—and very obvious in others. If each reader can understand that within every person with dementia there is a person alive inside, then I have done my job. If some recognize that threads of the person's life experiences provide avenues into that inner world of the person with dementia, then I have succeeded at achieving a new level of awareness for those readers. Stress levels will go down. Joy will replace some of the sadness that fills each day. Relationships can achieve new levels of understanding or quality. The health of caregivers will improve. In a world where a "dementia consciousness" will become pervasive, life will be filled with options for how it is impacts the lives of individuals and their families. For those who still do not understand what the phrase "dementia consciousness" means, I offer this simple explanation. "Dementia consciousness" is an expression of the human spirit through the altered lens of a human brain. This altered lens is shaped by the neurological changes of a brain disease or traumatic brain injury. Over time communications with that human spirit will shift away from the head toward the heart. New relationship opportunities will emerge.

♪

Every person has a life force that gives them the energy to go out into the world each day. Some people call that life force a soul. Others call it spirit. Still others have their own unique name for that life force. Different cultures and religions around the world lay claim to its origins. Everyone has a belief system that helps them to understand and explain what happens to that "life force" when it leaves the human body. No one system is better than another. Simply, each system has evolved over time and allows its followers to make sense of the everyday world.

For those with a condition or disease that creates dementia, that life force provides a vehicle for communication that most people do not recognize. After the normal channels of communication have been altered or lost completely due to damage to the brain, there are many venues still open to them. Increasingly people are beginning to recognize the gift of music and its ability to penetrate the wall between the inner world of the person with dementia and the outside world. As you have seen in the preceding pages, there are many other avenues available for you to travel—if you choose to go down those pathways.

Over time as technologies evolve and new ways of establishing lines of communication become available, we will witness new lines opening up to those with dementia that never existed. Along with these new technologies, I believe, we will see new treatments for the diseases that create a dementia process. Some of those diseases will be eradicated. Others will become less taxing on our families and society. Until that happens, I hope persons with dementia will achieve a new level of respect and attention among friends and families as well as their individual communities.

ACKNOWLEDGEMENTS

Without the encouragement and support of my cousins, James "Jimmy" Clodfelter, J.D. and Myrna Clodfelter Davis, this book would not have been written. I can never thank you enough!

My dear friend, Alan DeValle, helped me to stay on track and remain focused during this writing process. He always seemed to be there with words of support every time I wanted to give up. He is an angel!

Dr. Linda Blazina andABstract. David Morris are responsible for the additions of the Chemobrain material and the open heart surgery cognitive problems. They are each gifted clinicians and very dear friends. I am so grateful for them and their contributions to my life.

Tony Edens and his literary and legal wisdom and friendship across the years have a value that is somewhere beyond incalculable! His lessons on creating win-win relationships will be cherished forever.

Thanks go to my great nieces and nephews Madison, Brandon, and Bryson Trammell and Cayden and Carlisle Ward, for keeping me real and reminding me that life needs to be lived in the moment! I look forward to a future of watching them grow into exceptional adults with the unique skills and talents they each bring to the world!

To my Create Space team, thank you for your support during the production of this book. I especially want to thank my editor for his guidance and sweet comments.

Thank you Michael for giving me the opportunity to write books!

END NOTES

Introduction

1. Rohra, H. (2011). "A review of the ADI Meeting from a mind touched by dementia." *Alzheimer's Disease International Newsletter: Global Perspective.* March, p. 10.

Chapter One

Written permission for the use the stories referenced in this chapter was obtained by each individual prior to their use.

Chapter Two

2. American Psychiatric Association. (2010). *Diagnostic and Statistical Manual of Mental Disorders* (4th ed., text revision). Arlington, VA: American Psychiatric Association, pp. 147–171.
3. University of California Los Angeles. (2006). "Scientists find chemobrain no figment of the imagination." *Science Digest.* May 15, 2012.
4. Benedict, R. (1994). "Cognitive function after open-heart surgery: Are post-operative neuropsychological deficits caused by cardio-pulmonary bypass?" *Neuropsychological Review.* September, 4 (3) pp. 223–255.
5. *Dorland's Illustrated Medical Dictionary* (28th ed.). (1994). Philadelphia, PA: W. B. Saunders Co., pp. 439.
6. Rubins, P. (Ed.). (2011). *Guide to Understanding Dementia: Special Report.* Baltimore, MD: The Johns Hopkins School of Medicine, p. 2.
7. Albert, M., Rubins, P. (Ed.). (2011). "Mild cognitive impairments: Signs of early cognitive damage." *The Johns Hopkins Bulletins: Memory Disorders.* Fall Issue, pp. 4–10.

8. Albert, M., DeKosky, S., Dickson, D.; Dubois, S.; Feldman, H., Fox, N., Gamst, A., Holtzman, D., Jagust, W., Peterson, R., Snyder, P. (2010). *Criteria for Mild Cognitive Impairment Due to Alzheimer's Disease.* Special Report.
9. American Psychological Association. (2012). "Guidelines for the evaluation of dementia and age-related cognitive change." *American Psychologist.* Vol. 67, No. 1, pp. 1–9.
10. "Mild cognitive impairment: A comprehensive overview." (2011). MayoClinic.com, October 14.
11. Summit, P. (2011). "Pat Summit has early onset dementia." Open Letter to University of Tennessee, August 25.
12. Newcomb, A. (2011). "Glen Campbell reveals he has Alzheimer's." Press release. ABC News, June 22.
13. Reisenberg, B. (2011). "Seven stages of Alzheimer's." Chicago, IL: Alzheimer's Disease Association, October 27.
14. Lewy Body Dementia Association. (2012). "What is LBD?" Fact sheet. Lilburn, GA: Lewy Body Dementia Association.
15. Hershey, L., Olszewski, W., Morris, J. (ed). (1994). "Ischemic vascular dementia." *Handbook of Dementing Illnesses.* New York, NY: Marcel Dekker, Inc.
16. Reichman, W. (1994). "Non-degenerative dementing disorders." In C. Caffey, J. Cummings (Eds.). *Textbook of Geriatric Neuropsychiatry.* Washington, DC: American Psychiatric Press, Inc., pp. 370–376.
17. Alzheimer's Disease Association. (2011). "Vascular dementia: Fact sheet." Chicago, IL: Alzheimer's Disease Association.
18. Ibid.
19. Ibid.

20. The Michael J. Fox Foundation for Parkinson's Research. (2012). Fact sheet on Parkinson's disease. New York, NY: The Michael J. Fox Foundation for Parkinson's Research.
21. Ibid.
22. Brandt, J. (2011). "Parkinson's disease, cognitive impairment and dementia." *The John's Hopkins Bulletins: Memory Disorders.* Summer Issue, pp. 23–40.
23. Wojcieszek, J., Lang, A. (1994). "Hyperkinetic movement disorders." In C. Caffey, J. Cummings (Eds.). *Textbook of Geriatric Neuropsychiatry.* Washington, DC: American Psychiatric Association Press, Inc., pp. 411–415.
24. Sharma, T., Thomas, R. (2012). "Frontotemporal dementia initially misdiagnosed as a psychotic disorder: A case report." *Psychiatric Weekly.* Vol. 7, Issue 2, January 23.
25. LaMarre, A., Kramer, J. (2011). "Update on frontotemporal dementia." *National Academy of Neuropsychology Bulletin.* Vol. 26, No. 1, pp. 6–11.
26. Ibid. p. 7.
27. Ibid. pp. 7-8.
28. "A picture of Pick's disease from the inside out." (2011). *Dementia & Azheimer's Weekly Newsletter.* July 15, 2011.
29. First, M. (Ed.). (2010). "Post-concussion disorder." *Diagnostic and Statistical Manual of Mental Disorders* (4th ed., text revision). Washington, DC: American Psychiatric Association Press, Inc., pp. 760–762.
30. Johnson, V., Stewart, W., Smith, D. (2012). "Widespread tau and amyloid-beta pathology many years after a single traumatic brain injury in humans." *Brain Pathology.* Vol. 22, pp. 142–149.

End Notes

31. Tanielian, T., Jaycox, L. (Eds.) (2008). *Invisible Wounds of War: Psychological and Cognitive Injuries, Their Consequences and Services to Assist Recovery.* Los Angeles, CA: Rand Corporation.

32. National Center for Injury Prevention and Control. (2003) *Report to Congress on Mild Traumatic Brain Injury in the United States: Steps to Prevent a Serious Public Health Problem.* Atlanta, GA: Centers for Disease Control and Prevention.

33. Centers for Disease Control and Prevention (2009). "Prevalence and most common causes of disability among adults – United States, 2005." *MMWR.* Vol. 58, Issue 16, pp. 421–426.

34. Hummer, S. (2012). "Hard knocks toll: Former placers claim the NFL concealed the long term costs of repeated hits to the head." *Atlanta Journal Constitution.* January 29, Section C, pp. 1, *Atlanta Journal Constitution.* January 29, Section C, pp. 1, 8.

35. McKee, A., Cantu, R., Nowinski, A., Headly-White, E., Gavett, B., Budson, A., Santini, V., Lee, H., Kubilus, C., Stern, R. (2009). "Chronic traumatic encephalopathy in athletes: Progressive tauopathy following repetitive head injury." *Journal of Neuropathology/Experimental Neurology.* Vol. 68, Issue 7, pp. 709–735.

36. Cantor, J. (2008). "Improving the recognition and treatment of traumatic brain injury." *Psychiatric Weekly.* Vol. 3, No. 12, March 24.

37. Neutal, D. (2012). "Concussions hit teens worse than adults, young children: Research." *Vancouver Sun.* February 28.

38. Downs, D. Abwender, D. (2002). "Neuropsychological impairment in soccer athletes." *Journal of Sports Medicine and Physical Fitness.* Vol. 42 No. 1, March, pp. 103–107.

39. Ances, B., Ellis, R. (2007). "Dementia and neurocognitive disorders due to HIV-1 infection." *Seminars in Neurology.* Vol. 27, No. 1, February, pp. 86–92.
40. Casanova-Sotolongo, P.; Casanova-Carrillo, P.; Casanova-Carrillo, C. (2002). "Dementia associated with AIDS." *Revue Neurologigue* (Paris). Vol. 34, No. 8, April 16–30, pp. 781 – 787.
41. Gray, F. (1998). "Dementia and human immunodeficiency virus infection." *Revue Neurologigue.* (Paris) 154, Supplement 2: S91–98.
42. Woods, S., Moore, D., Weber, E., Grant, I. (2009). "Cognitive neuropsychology of HIV-associated neurocognitive disorders." *Neuropsychological Review.* Vol. 19, Issue 2, June, pp. 152–168.
43. Grant, I.; Atkinson, J. (1995). "Psychiatric aspects of immune deficiency syndrome." In H. Kaplan & B. Sadock (Eds.). *Comprehensive Textbook of Psychiatry* (Vol. 2). Baltimore, MD: Williams & Wilkins, pp. 1644–1669.
44. Antinori, A., Arendt, G., Becker, J., Brew, B., Byrd, D., Cherner, M. (2007). "Updated research nosology for HIV associated neurocognitive disorders." *Neurology.* Vol. 69, pp. 1789–1799.
45. Robertson, K., Smurzynski, M., Parsons, T., Wu, K., Bosch, R., Wu, J. (2007). "The prevalence and incidence of neurocognitive impairment in HARRT era." *AIDS.* Vol. 21, pp. 1915–1921.
46. Goodkin, K., Wilkie, F., Concha, M., Hinkins, C., Symes, S., Baldewicz, T. (2001). "Aging and neuro-AIDS conditions and the changing spectrum of HIV-1 associated morbidity and mortality." *Journal of Clinical Epidemiology.* Vol. 54 (12 Supplement 1), S35–43.

47. Grant, I., Atkinson, J. (1999). "Neuropsychiatric aspects of HIV infection and AIDS." In B. Sadock & V. Sadock (Eds.) *Kaplan and Sadock's Comprehensive Textbook of Psychiatry*. Baltimore, MD: Williams & Wilkins, pp. 308–335.
48. Grant, I., Sacktor, N., McArthur, J. (2005). "HIV neurocognitive disorders." In H. Gendelman, I. Grant, I. Eversall, S. Lipton, & S. Swindells (Eds.) *The Neurology of AIDS* (2nd ed.). New York, NY: Oxford University Press, pp. 359–373.
49. Alisky, J. (2007). "The coming problem of HIV associated Alzheimer's disease." *Medical Hypothesis*. Vol. 65, No. 5, pp. 1140–1143.
50. University of California Los Angeles. (2006). "Scientists find "chemo-brain" no figment of the imagination." *Science Daily*. October 6.
51. Wefel, J., Lenzi, R., Theriault, R., Buzdar. A., Cruickshank, S., Meyers, C. (2004). "Chemobrain in breast carcinoma?: A prologue." *Cancer*. Vol. 101, No. 3, August 1, pp. 466–475.
52. Schagen, S., vanDam, F., Muller, M., Boogerd, W., Lindeboom, J., Bruning P. (1999). "Cognitive deficits after postoperative adjunctive chemotherapy for breast carcinoma." *Cancer*. Vol. 85, No. 3, February 1, pp. 640–650.
53. Schagen, S., Hamburger, H., Muller, M., Boogerd, W., vanDam, F. (2001). "Neuropsychological evaluation of late effects of adjuvant high-dose chemotherapy on cognitive function." *Journal of Neuro-Oncology*. Vol. 51, No. 2, January, pp. 159–165.
54. Falleti, M., Sanfilippo, A., Maruff, P., Weih, L., Phillips, K. (2005). "The nature and severity of cognitive impairment associated with adjuvant chemotherapy in women with breast cancer:

A meta-analysis of the current literature." *Brain Cognition.* Vol. 59, No. 1, October, pp. 60–70.

55. Vodermaire, A. (2009). "Breast cancer treatment and cognitive function: The current state of evidence underlying mechanisms and potential treatments." *Women's Health (London England).* Vol. 5, No. 5, September, pp. 503–516.

56. University of Rochester Medical Center (2009). "Chemo's toxicity to brain revealed, possible treatment identified." *Science Daily.* December 17.

57. Syrjala, K., Artherholt, S., Kurland, B., Langer, S., Roth-Roemer, S., Elrod, J., Dikmen, S. (2011). "Prospective neurocognitive function over 5 years after allogenic hematopoietic cell transplantation for cancer survivors compared with matched controls at 5 years." *Journal of Clinical Oncology.* Vol. 29, No. 17, pp. 2397–2404.

58. Walzer, T.; Hermann, M. (1998). "Neuropsychological and psychopathologic changes following cardiac surgical procedures." *Fortschr Neurol & Psychiatry.* Vol. 66, No. 2, February, pp. 68–83.

59. Benedict, R. (1994). "Cognitive function after open – heart surgery: Are post-operative neuropsychological deficits caused by Cardiopulmonary bypass?" *Neuropsychological Review.* Vol. 4, No. 3, September, pp. 223–255.

60. DiCarlo, A., Perna, A., Pantoni, L., Basile, A., Bonacchi, M., Pracucci, G., Trelfoloni, G., Brancco, L. Sangiovanni, V., Piccini, C., Plamarini, M., Caroneeto, F., Biondi, E., Sani, G., Inzitari, D. (2001). "Clinically relevant cognitive impairment after cardiac surgery: A 6 month follow-up study." *Journal of Neurological Science.* Vol. 188, No. 1-2, July 5, pp. 85–93.

61. Ebert, A.; Walzer, T.; Huth, C.; Hermann, M. (2001). "Early neuro-behavioral disorders after cardiac surgery: A comparative analysis of coronary artery bypass graft surgery and valve replacement." *Journal of Cardiothoracic Vascular Anesthesia.* Vol. 15, No. 1, February pp. 15–19.
62. Mehta, Y., Singh. R. (2010). "Cognitive dysfunction after cardiac surgery." *Journal of Alzheimer's Disease.* Vol. 22, Supplement 3, pp. 115–120.
63. Teixeira-Sousa, V., Costa, C., Costa, A., Grangeia, R., Reis, C., Coelho, R. (2008) "Neurocognitive dysfunction after valve surgery." *Acta Medicine Portugal* Vol. 21, No. 5, September–October, pp. 475–482.
64. Alzheimer's Disease Association (2012). "Alzheimer's disease facts and Figures." Chicago, IL: Alzheimer's Disease Association. March 11.

Chapter Three

65. Aldrige, D. (1993). "Is there evidence for spiritual healing?" *Advances: The Journal of Mind-Body Health.* Vol. 9, No. 4. pp. 4–21.
66. Kuhn, C. (1988). "A spiritual inventory of the medically ill patient." *Psychiatric Medicine.* 6: pp. 87–100.
67. Forrest, D., Richmond, C. (2000). *Symphony of Spirits: Encounters with the Spiritual Dimensions of Alzheimer's.* New York, NY: St. Martin's Press.
68. Ibid. pp. 71–76.
69. Kübler-Ross, E., Kessler, D. (1969). *On Death and Dying.* New York, NY: MacMillan Publishing Company. 70. Paragament, K., Sweeny, P. (2011). "Building spiritual fitness in the army." *American Psychologist.* Vol. 66, No. 1, pp. 58–64.

71. Ibid. pp. 58.
72. Ibid. pp 58–59.
73. Ibid. pp. 59
74. Ibid. pp. 59.
75. Private Conversation with Native American Elder. (2001). Knoxville, TN.
76. Ellis, N. (1988). *Awakening Osiris: The Egyptian Book of the Dead*. Grand Rapids, MI; Phones Press.
77. Ibid. pp. 23.
78. Ibid. pp. 24.
79. Garland, E., Frederickson, B., Kring, A., Johnson, D., Meyer, P, Penn, D. (2010). "Upward spirals of positive emotions counter downward spirals of negativity: Insights from the broad-and-build theory and affective neuroscience on the treatment of emotion dysfunctions and deficits in psychopathology." *Clinical Psychology Review*. Vol. 30, pp. 849–864.
80. Frederickson, R., Cohn, M., Coffey, K., Pek, J., Finkel, S. (2008). "Open hearts build lives: Positive emotions induced through loving kindness, mediation build consequential personal resources." *Journal of Personality and Social Psychology*. Vol. 95, No. 5, pp. 1045–1062.

Chapter Four
81. Moore, T. (2011). "Spirituality and care of the soul in psychotherapy." Presentation at the New England Educational Institute, Santa Fe, NM, October 21–24.
82. Sacks, O. (2009). "Alzheimer's and the power of music." *Dementia and Alzheimer's Weekly*. October 18–25.
83. Jacobs, B. (2007). "Reaching Alzheimer's through music." In O.

Sacks (Ed.) <u>Musciophilia: Tales of Music and the Brain.</u> New York, NY: Alfred A. Knopf.
84. Watkins, K. (2001). "Singing and laughing: Good medicine." *OUTLOOK: A Periodical About Brain Injury.* Vol. 2, Issue 1, p. 23.
85. Levitin, D. (2007). *This Is Your Brain On Music: The Science of Human Obsession.* New York, NY: Plume/Penguin.
86. Ibid.
87. Watkins, K. (2001). "Singing and laughing: Good medicine." *OUTLOOK: A Periodical About Brain Injury.* Vol. 2, Issue 1, p. 23.
88. Wilson, M. (2010). "Dementia patients paint what they can't say." *Silicon Valley Community Newspapers.* March 9.
89. Jarvis, J. (2008). "Art cuts through the fog of Alzheimer's." *The Fort Worth Star Telegram, p. 2*
90. Forrest, D.; Richmond, C. (2000). *Symphony of Spirits: Encounters with the Spiritual Dimensions of Alzheimer's.* New York, NY: St. Martin's Press.
91. Abrahms, S. (2012). "A comfort-and-joy approach." *AARP Bulletin.* July–August, p. 14.92. Edwards, N., Beck, A. (2002). "Animal-assisted therapy and nutrition in Alzheimer's disease." *Western Journal of Nursing Research.* Vol. 24, No. 6, pp. 697–712.
93. Kappeter, I. (2012). "Intergenerational activities." *Alzheimer's Disease International Newsletter.* Vol. 22, No. 2, p. 8.
94. Valnet, J. (2005). "Aroma therapy and the 4 'A' of Alzheimer's." *Geriatrics and Aging: Nonpharmacological Management of Agitated Behaviors Associated With Dementia.* Vol. 8, No. 4, pp. 26–30.

95. *The Practice of Aroma Therapy.* (1990). Rochester, VT: Healing Arts Press.
96. Alzheimer's Disease International (2010) "Forward." *Alzheimer's Disease International Report 2010: The Global Economic Impact of Dementia: Executive Summary.* London: Alzheimer's Disease International, p. 1.
97. Ibid. p. 3.
98. Alzheimer's Disease International Member's Forum Hong Kong SAR (2011). "Helping children spot the signs of dementia." *Alzheimer's Disease International Newsletter.* Vol. 21, No. 2, p. 6.
99. Spitzer, P. (2008). "Laughter Boss: Introducing a new position in aged care." In B. Warren (Ed.) *Using the Creative Arts in Healthcare and Therapy.* London: Routledge.
100. Westberg, N. (2003). "Hope, laughter and humor in residents and staff at an assisted living facility." *Journal of Mental Health Counseling.* Vol. 25, No. 1, pp. 16–32.
101. Low, L. (2011). "Humor may be the best medicine for agitated dementia Patients." *Senior Journal.* September 21.
102. "Humor as effective as medication in treating agitation in dementia." (2011). *Science Daily.* September 21.
103. Zeiss, A. Kasl-Godley, J. (2001). "Sexuality in older adult relationships." *Generations.* Vol. 25, No. 2, pp. 18–25.
104. Davies, H., Newkirk, L., Pitts, C., Coughlin, C., Sridhar, S., Zeiss, L., Zeiss, A. (2010). "The impact of dementia and mild memory impairment (MMI) on intimacy and sexuality in spousal relationships." *International Psychogeriatrics.* Vol. 22, pp. 618–628.
105. Moore, K. (2010). "Sexuality and sense of self in later life: Japanese men's and women's reflections on sex and aging." *Journal of Cross-Cultural Gerontology.* Vol. 25, No. 2, pp. 149–163.

106. Davis, H., Zeiss, A., Tinklenberg, J. (1998). "Sexuality and intimacy in Alzheimer's patients and their partners." *Sexuality and Disability*. Vol. 16, No. 3, p. 193–203.
107. Sharpe, T. (2004). "Introduction to sexuality in later life." The Family Journal. Vol. 12, No. 2, pp. 199–205.
108. Bamford, S. (2011). "The last taboo: Dementia, sexuality, intimacy and sexual behavior in care homes." *Alzheimer's Disease International Newsletter*. Vol. 21, No. 4, p. 8.

Chapter Five

109. O'Bryant, S., Xiao, B., Huebinger, R., Wilhelmsen, K., Edwards, M., Graff-Radford, N., Doody, R., Diaz-Arrastia, R. (2011). "A blood-based tool for Alzheimer's disease that spans and plasma: Findings from TARC and ADNI." *PLoS ONE*. Vol. 6, No. 12.
110. Sabbagh, M., Malek-Ahmadi, M., Kataria, R., Belden, C., Conner, D., Pearson, C., Jacobson, S., Davis, K., Yaari, R., Singh, U. (2010). "The Alzheimer's questionnaire: A proof of concept study for a new informant-based dementia assessment." *Journal of Alzheimer's Disease*. Vol. 22, No. 3, pp. 1015–1021.
111. O'Bryant, S., Xiao, G., Barber, R., Reisch, J., Doody, R., Fairchild, T., Adams, P., Waring, S., Diaz-Arrastia, R. (2010). "A serum protein based algorithm for the detection of Alzheimer's disease." *Archives of Neurology*. Vol. 167, pp. 1077–1081.
112. Eli Lilly and Company (2012). "FDA approves amyloid (Florbetapir) F 18 Injection for use in patients being evaluated for Alzheimer's disease and other causes of cognitive decline." Press release. Indianapolis, IN, April 6.
113. Rafii, M. (2012). "Bexarotene in context: A look at the exciting

results." *Alzheimer's Disease Information Network ADIN Monthly Newsletter.* No. 40, March, pp. 1–2.
114. Kamel, H., Navi, B., Fahimi, J. (2012). "National trends in ambulance use by patients with stroke, 1997–2008." *Journal of American Medical Association.* Vol. 307, No. 10, March 14, pp. 1026–1028.
115. Woods, S., Moore, D., Weber, E., Grant, I. (2009). "Cognitive neuropsychology of HIV-Associated neurocognitive disordes." *Neuropsychology Review.* Vol. 19 , No. 2, June, pp. 152–168.
116. Chen, Y. (2012). "HIV treatment as prevention: 2011's scientific breakthrough of the year." Seattle Cancer Care Alliance's *QUEST Magazine,* Seattle, WA.
117. Rubins, P. (Ed.). (2012). "Forgetfulness, confusion and disorientation—symptoms of chemobrain." *The Johns Hopkins Health Alerts: Memory.* February 20.
118. Cleveland Clinic (2012). "The effects of bypass surgery on neurological function." *Fact Sheet On Cardiovascular Disease & Neurological Function.* Cleveland, Ohio.
119. Associated Press (2012). "Mega-suit rips NFL on head injuries." Philadelphia, PA, June 7.
120. Neutel, D. (2012). "Concussions hit teens worse than adults, young children: Research." *Vancouver Sun.* February 28.
121. Baillargeon, A., Lassonde, M., Leclerc, S., Ellemberg, D. (2012). "Neurological and neurophysiological assessment of sports concussions in children, adolescents and adults." *Brain Injury.* Vol. 26, No. 3, pp. 211–220.
122. Henry, L., Tremblay, J., Tremblay, S., Lee, A., Brun, C., Lepore, N., Theoret, H., Ellemberg, D., Lassonde, M. (2011). "Acute and chronic changes in diffusivity measure after sports

concussion. *Journal of Neurotrauma.* Vol. 10, October 28, pp. 2049–2059.

123. Henry, L., Tremblay, S., Leclerc, S., Khiat, A., Boulanger, Y., Ellemberg, D., Lassonde, M. (2011). "Metabolic changes in concussed American football players during the acute and chronic post-injury phases." *BMC Neurology.* Vol. 11, August 23, pp. 105.

124. "Treating veterans will cost at least $5 billion by 2020 Congressional Budget Office says." (2011). *Monitor on Psychology.* November, p. 11.

125. Cantor, J. (2008). "Improving the recognition and treatment of traumatic brain injury." *Psychiatric Weekly.* Vol. 3, Issue 12, March 24.

126. Carper, J. (2010). *100 Simple Things You Can Do to Prevent Alzheimer's and Age-Related Memory Loss.* New York, NY: Little Brown and Company.

127. Song, X., Mitnitksi, A., Rockwood, K. (2011). "Non-traditional risk factors combine to predict Alzheimer's disease and dementia." *Neurology.* Vol. 77, No. 3, July 19, pp. 227–234.

128. Rabins, P. (Ed.). (2011). "Memory boosters." *The Johns Hopkins Medicine Special Report: The Memory Bulletin*, pp. 1-6.

Chapter Six

129. Alzheimer's Disease Association. (2012). *Unpaid caregivers: 2012 Alzheimer's Disease Facts and Figures.* Chicago, IL: Alzheimer's Disease Association.

130. Pennebaker, J., Kiecolt-Glaser, J., Kiecolt-Glaser, R. (1988). "Disclosure of traumas and immune function: Health implications for psychotherapy." *Journal of Consulting and Clinical Psychology.* Vol. 56, pp. 239–245.

131. Pennebaker, J. (1997). *Opening Up: The Healing Power of Expressing Emotion.* New York, NY; Guilford Press.
132. Pennebaker, J. (1997). "Writing about emotional experiences as a therapeutic process." *Psychological Science.* Vol. 8, pp. 162–166.
133. Petrie, K., Booth, R., Pennebaker, J. (1998). "The immunological effects if thought suppression." *Journal of Personality and Social Psychology.* Vol. 75, pp. 1264–1272.

Chapter Seven

134. World Health Organization & Alzheimer's Disease International. (2012). *Dementia: A Public Health Priority.* Press Release. London: World Health Organization & Alzheimer's Disease International.
135. Alzheimer's Disease International. (1999). "Caring for people with dementia around the world." Fact Sheet 5. London: Alzheimer's Disease International, June.
136. Nagamatsu, L., Handy, T., Hsu, L., Voss, M., Liu-Ambrose, T. (2012). "Resistance training promotes cognitive and functional brain plasticity in seniors with probable mild cognitive impairment." *Archives of Internal Medicine.* Vol., 172, No. 8, pp. 666–668.
137. Devore, E.; Kang, J., Breteler, M., Grodstein, F. (2012). "Dietary intakes of berries and flavonoids in relation to cognitive decline." *Annals of Neurology.* April 25.
138. deMendoca, A.; Cunhn, R. (2010). "Therapeutic opportunities for caffeine in Alzheimer's disease and other neurodegenerative disorders." *Journal of Alzheimer's Disease.* Vol. 20, Supplement 1, pp. S1-2.
139. Arendash, C., Cao, O. (2010). "Caffeine and coffee as therapeutics against Alzheimer's disease." *Journal of Alzheimer's Disease.* Vol. 20, Supplement 1, pp. S117–126.

140. Chen, X., Ghribi, O., Geiger, J. (2010). "Caffeine protects against disruptions of the blood-brain barrier in animal models of Alzheimer's and Parkinson's diseases." *Journal of Alzheimer's Disease.* Vol. 20, Supplement 1, pp. S127–141.

141. Suchy, J., Lee, S., Ahmed, A., Shea, T. (2010). "Dietary supplementation with pecans delays motor neuron pathology in transgenic mice expressing G93A mutant human superoxide dimuse-1." *Current Topics in Nutraceutical Research.* Vol. 8, No. 1, pp. 45–54.

142. Newport, M. (2011). *Alzheimer's Disease: What if There Was a Cure? The Story of Ketones.* Clearwater, FL: Basic Health Publications.

143. Krikorion, R., Shidler, M., Dangelo, K., Couch, S., Benoit, S., Clegg, D. (2012). "Dietary ketosis enhances memory in mild cognitive impairment." *Neurobiology of Aging.* Vol. 33, No. 2. pp. 425.

144. Gordon, M. (2008). *The Clinical Applications of Interventional Endocrinology.* Encino, CA: Phoenix Books & Millennium Health Centers, Inc.

145. "Scientists find anti-Alzheimer's gene mutation." (2012). Press release. Yahoo – ABC News Network, July 12.

146. Verghese, J., Lipton, R., Katz, M., Hall, C., Derby, C., Luslansky, G., Ambrose, A., Silwinsky, M., Buschke, H. (2003). Leisure activities and the risk of dementia in the elderly." *New England Journal of Medicine,* Vol. 348, pp. 2508-2516.

147. Davies, P. (2012). "Crosswords, computers and cognition: What's going on in your Brain?" Invited Speaker, Twenty-Fifth Annual Meeting of New York Alzheimer's Association, October 17.

APPENDIX
"Seven Stages of Alzheimer's"

Stage One: There are no symptoms. The person does not experience any memory problems. This stage is put here to make sure the public understands that Alzheimer's disease begins its destructive processes years before there are any signs or symptoms present.

Stage Two: The person may feel like she has some memory lapses or "senior moments." She/he may forget familiar words or the location of everyday objects. No symptoms of dementia can be detected during a doctor's exam. There is evidence of very mild cognitive decline, which may be normal age-related changes or the very earliest signs of Alzheimer's disease. This is a hard stage for everyone.

Stage Three: Mild cognitive or mental decline is evident. Family, friends, and or co-workers begin to notice subtle difficulties. The person with the problem has no recognition of any problems. She/he will deny having any problems. During a visit to the doctor's office, the doctor *may* be able to detect problems in memory or concentration. Common problems seen here include:

- Noticeable problems coming up with the right word or name
- Trouble remembering names when introduced to new people
- Having noticeably greater difficulty performing tasks in social or work settings. Forgetting material that she/he has just read
- Losing or misplacing a valuable object, like a wallet, car keys, or a checkbook
- Increasing trouble with planning or organizing

Stage Four: A moderate decline in cognitive functions—the ability to think and remember things—is seen. The person is now viewed as having the mild or early-stage of Alzheimer's disease. During an office visit the doctor who uses a careful medical interview *should be able to detect clear-cut* symptoms of Alzheimer's. These will include such things as:
- Forgetting recent events
- Impaired ability to perform challenging mental arithmetic, like counting backwards from 100 by sevens
- Greater problems with performing complex tasks, such as planning dinner for guests, making a trip to the store to buy groceries, cooking a meal on the stove, paying bills, or managing finances
- Forgetting about one's own personal history
- Becoming moody or withdrawn, especially in socially or mentally challenging situations

Stage Five: Signs of moderately severe cognitive decline become clear. The person now has moderate or mid-stage of Alzheimer's. There are clear gaps in the individual's memory and thinking abilities. She/he will begin to need help with day-to-day activities. Signs of the progression of the disease at this point include:

- Cannot recall/remember her/his own address or telephone number or the high school or college from which she/he graduated
- Gets confused about where she/he or what day it is
- Has trouble with less challenging mental arithmetic such as counting backward from forty by subtracting by fours
- Needs help choosing proper clothing for the season or the occasion
- Still remembers significant details about her/himself and family members
- Is still able to feed her/himself and use the toilet without assistance

*Stage Six: S*evere cognitive decline is seen. This is the *moderately severe or mid-stage* of Alzheimer's. The person's memory continues to worsen. Personality changes may take place. The person may become paranoid, hostile, angry, and aggressive, or docile, pleasant, and cooperative. (This is the hardest time for caregivers.) The person will begin to need extensive help every day with such things as dressing her/himself, bathing, shaving, mouth care, hair care, toileting, food and meal preparation and clean up, and the preparation and delivery of all medications taken and purchased. Caregivers can begin to expect the person to show one or more of these signs:

- Lose awareness of recent experiences as well as her/his surroundings

- Remember her/his own name but have trouble recalling her/his own personal history
- Be able to distinguish between familiar and unfamiliar faces but has trouble remembering the name of a spouse or caregiver. The person will "shadow" the spouse or partner she/he has known for years—following behind him or her everywhere.
- Will need help dressing properly and may make mistakes such as putting on pajamas over daytime clothes or shoes on the wrong feet, undergarments on top of daytime wear, or multiple layers of the same type of clothing or any combination of the above
- Have major changes in sleep patterns: sleeping during the day and becoming restless at night and roaming throughout the night. If this behavior goes on for three or more days, the person will usually become psychotic and require hospitalization to re-stabilize her/his sleep patterns
- Will need help with the details of toileting (such as wiping the buttocks and disposing of the tissue properly and flushing the toilet). These skills become lost and/or forgotten. No amount of reminders will change the behaviors!
- Will have increasingly frequent trouble controlling her/his bladder and bowels. The use of adult diapers will usually be required
- Display major personality and behavioral changes. These can include suspiciousness and delusions (such as believing that her/his caregiver is an imposter or the caregiver has stolen her/his wallet and all of her/his money). Other common changes you might see include compulsive, repetitive behaviors like hand-wringing, tearing tissue paper, or stuffing clothes in

the toilet. On some occasions the person may believe another person is her/his lover or spouse. This can be especially difficult for family members
- A tendency to wander out of the house and/or become lost. In some states there are now "Silver Alerts" to notify the public of a missing senior with dementia

Stage Seven: Very severe cognitive decline is evident. The person is in the severe or late-stage of Alzheimer's. In this final stage, the person loses the ability to recognize or respond to her/his surroundings. She/he is unable to carry on a conversation with anyone—including the spouse or partner. Eventually, the individual is unable to control all movements. Speech will be made up of only a single word or a few phrases. Help with all personal care is required; this includes eating and using the toilet. Loss of the ability to smile or sit up without support or even hold her/his head up may occur. All of the person's reflexes become abnormal. Swallowing becomes impaired. Gagging is common. Muscles become rigid. Urinary tract infections as well as respiratory infections are common. In the end, one or the other of these infections usually becomes fatal.

Lewy Body Dementia

Symptoms of LBD include:

1. Problems with memory, problem solving, planning, and abstract or analytical thinking.
2. Cognitive Fluctuations involve unpredictable changes in concentration and attention from day to day.
3. Parkinson's like symptoms include rigidity or stiffness, shuffling gait, tremor and slowness of movement.
4. Auditory and/or Visual hallucinations may be present. If they are not disruptive, no treatment is warranted. If they are frightening or dangerous, medical treatment should be obtained.
5. REM Sleep Disorder (RBD) involves acting out dreams – sometimes violently. If this problem exists, medical treatment should be obtained.
6. Other symptoms that will need to be monitored and treated include:
    a. Temperature regulation and blood pressure levels.
    b. Dizziness & fainting
    c. Sensitivity to heat and cold
    d. Sexual dysfunction
    e. Urinary incontinence or constipation
    f. Falls
    g. Excessive sleepiness or transient loss of consciousness
    h. Mood disorders such as depression or delusions

Lewy Body Dementia Association, 2012

APPENDIX

Post-Concussion Syndrome

Post-concussion syndrome is a complex disorder in which a variable combination of post-concussion symptoms—such as headaches and dizziness—last for weeks and sometimes months after the injury that caused the concussion.

Concussion is a mild traumatic brain injury, usually occurring after a blow to the head. Loss of consciousness isn't required for a diagnosis of concussion or post-concussion syndrome. In fact, the risk of post-concussion syndrome doesn't appear to be associated with the severity of the initial injury.

In most people, post-concussion syndrome symptoms occur within the first seven to 10 days and go away within three months, though they can persist for a year or more. Post-concussion syndrome treatments are aimed at easing specific symptoms.

Post-concussion symptoms include:
- Dizziness
- Fatigue
- Headaches
- Irritability
- Anxiety
- Insomnia
- Loss of concentration and memory
- Noise and light sensitivity

Headaches that occur after a concussion can vary and may feel like tension-type headaches or migraine headaches. Most, however, are tension-type headaches, which may be associated with a neck injury that happened at the same time as the head injury. In some cases, people experience behavior or emotional changes after a mild traumatic brain injury. Family members may notice that the person has become more irritable, suspicious, argumentative or stubborn.

Mayo Clinic, 2012

RECOMMENDED READING

Take the next five or ten minutes to laugh yourself silly over the very thought of having *any extra time* to read another book. Once you are finished with that short boost to your immune system, take a few minutes to look over this list of books. There may be one or two that spark your interest.

Forrest, D. , Richmond, C. (2000). *Symphony of Spirits: Encounters with the Spiritual Dimensions of Alzheimer's.* New York, N.Y.: St. Martin's Press. ISBN: 0-312-24101-1

Kabat-Zinn, J., Davidson, R., Houshmand, Z. (2012). *The Mind's Own Physician: A Scientific Dialogue with the Dalai Lama on the Healing Power of Meditation.* Oakland, CA: New Harbinger Publications. ISBN-13: 978-1572249684

Krippner, S., Welch, P. (1992). *Spiritual Dimensions of Healing: From Native Shamanism to Contemporary Health Care.* New York, NY: Irvington Publishers, Inc. ISBN: 0-8290-3162-6

Kubler-Ross, E., Kessler, D. (2000). *Life Lessons: Two Experts on Death and Dying Teach Us About the Mysteries of Life and Living.* New York, NY: Scribner. ISBN: 0-684-87074-6

Laszio, E., Dennis, K. I. (Eds). (2012). *The New Science and Spirituality Reader.* Rochester, VT: Inner Traditions, Bear & Company. ISBN-13: 978-1-59477-476-8

Mace, N.L., Rubins, P. V. (1981). *The 36-Hour Day, Revised Edition: A Family Guide to Caring for Persons with Alzheimer's Disease, Related Dementing Illnesses, and Memory Loss in Later Life.* Baltimore, MD: The Johns Hopkins University Press. ISBN-13: 978-0801840340

Meindl, A. (2012). *At Left Brain Turn Right: An Uncommon Path to Shutting Up Your Inner Critic, Giving Fear the Finger and Having an Amazing Life.* Los Angeles, CA: Meta Creative. ISBN-13: 978-0615534862

Moore, T. (2010). *Care of the Soul in Medicine: Healing Guidance for Patients, Families, and the People who Care for Them.* Carlsbad, CA: Hay House, Inc. ISBN-13: 978-1401925642 *Dark Nights of the Soul: A Guide to Finding Your Way Through Life's Ordeals.* (2005). New York, NY. Gotham Books, Penguin Group Publisher. ISBN: 1-592-40067-1

Pearce, J.C. (2012). *The Heart-Mind Matrix: How the Heart Can Teach the Mind New Ways to Think.* Rochester, VT: Park Street Press/Bear & Company. ISBN-13: 978-1-59477-488-1

Scott, C. (2013). *Music and Its Secret Influence: Throughout the Ages.* Rochester, VT: Inner Traditions – Bear & Company. ISBN: 978-1-59477-487-4

Recommended Reading

Small, G., Vorgan, G. (2012). *The Alzheimer's Prevention Program: Keep Your Brain Healthy for the Rest of Your Life.* New York, NY: Workman Publishing. ISBN-13: 978-0-7611-6526-2

Tart, C. (Ed.). (1997). *Body, Mind, Spirit: Exploring the Parapsychology of Spirituality.* Charlottesville, VA: Hampton Roads Publishing Company, Inc. ISBN: 1-57174-073-2

ABOUT THE AUTHOR

Deborah A. Forrest, Ph.D., is a Registered Clinical Psychologist and a Registered Nurse. She earned her doctorate degree in clinical psychology at The Fielding Graduate Institute, Santa Barbara, California under the tutelage of Dr. Catherine Sanders, the late Dr. Elisabeth Kübler-Ross, and the late Dr. Inge Broverman. She completed a one-year postdoctoral fellowship in geriatric neuropsychology at the University of Kentucky. Her 2000 book, *Symphony of Spirits: Encounters with the Spiritual Dimensions of Alzheimer's,* was an international bestseller.

Share your own stories and experiences with Dr. Forrest @ www.drdeborahforrest.com

RESOURCES

The following pages contain information for people seeking assistance for a loved one with dementia living in another part of the USA or in a Foreign Country.

ALZHEIMER'S ASSOCIATIONS

Listed associations are members of Alzheimer's Disease International, except for those marked with *. Regional groups for Europe and Latin America are listed at the end of the section.

Albania *
Albanian Alzhiemer Society
Rr. Themistokli Germenji
Pall 10
Tirana
Albania
Tel/Fax: +355 4223 3289
Email: fleurapsy@yahoo.co.uk

Argentina
Asociación de Lucha contra el Mal de Alzheimer
Lacarra No 78
1407 Capital Federal, Buenos Aires
Argentina
Tel/Fax: +54 11 4671 1187
Email: info@alma-alzheimer.org.ar
Web: www.alma-alzheimer.org.ar

Armenia
Alzheimer's Disease Armenian Association
Prof Michail Aghajanov Phd
Head of the Biochemistry Dept.
Yerevan State Medical University
2 Koriun Str
Yerevan 375025
Armenia
Tel: + 3741 582 412
Fax: + 3741 589 219
Email: michail.aghajanov@meduni.am

Aruba
Fundacion Alzheimer Aruba (FAA)
Avenida Milo Croes 29, Suite C
Oranjestad
Aruba
Tel: +297 582 1684
Fax: +297 584 8416
Email: alzheimeraruba@gmail.com
Web: www.alzheimer-aruba.org

Australia
Alzheimer's Australia
P.O. Box 4019
Hawker
ACT 2614
Australia
Tel: +61 2 6254 4233

Helpline: 1800 100 500
Fax: +61 2 6278 7225
Web: www.fightdementia.org.au

Austria
Alzheimer Austria
Reisnerstrasse 41
1030 Vienna, Austria
Tel/Fax: +43 1 713 6208
Email: alzheimeraustria@aon.at
Web: www.alzheimer-selbsthilfe.at

Bahrain *
Alzheimer Support Group
Dr Adel Al-Offi
Psychiatric Hospital
P.O.Box 5128
Kingdom Of Bahrain
Tel: +973 17 279 326
Helpline:+973 39425525
Email: draaloffi@gmail.com

Bangladesh
Alzheimer Society of Bangladesh
Hall Para
PO:Thakurgaon-5100
Thakurgaon Sader
Bangladesh
Tel: +88 0172 049 8197
Email: alzbangladesh@yahoo.com

Barbados
Barbados Alzheimer's Association Inc
Room #3 Bethesda
Black Rock
St Michael
Barbados
Tel: +1 246 438 7111
Fax: +1 246 427 4256
Email: barbadosalzheimersassociation@caribsurf.com

Belgium
Ligue Nationale Alzheimer Liga
Rue Brogniezstraat, 46
B - 1070
Brussel - Bruxelles - Brussels
Helpline: (within Belgium) 0800 15 225
Email: info@alzheimer-belgium.be
Web: www.alzheimer-belgium.be

Bermuda
Alzheimer's Family Support Group
P.O.Box DV114
Devonshire DVBX
Bermuda
Tel: +441 238 2168 (pm)
Fax: +441 234 1765
Email: JulieKay@ibl.bm

Bolivia *
Asociación Boliviana de Alzheimer y Otras Demencias
Casilla No. 9302
La Paz
Bolivia
Tel: +591 2249 4143
Email: elvio904@gmail.com

Brazil
FEBRAZ - Federação Brasileira de Associaçãoes de Alzheimer
CF 542214 e o endereco
Rua Frei Caneca, 915
conjunto 2, Sao Paulo, Brazil
01307-003
Tel/Fax: +55 11 3237 0385
Helpline: 0 800 55 1906
Email: febrazbr@gmail.com

Bulgaria
Compassion Alzheimer Bulgaria
Tzanko Djustabanov 30, fl.3
9000 Varna
Bulgaria
Tel: +359 52 505 873
Fax: +359 52 505 873
Email: compassion.alz@abv.bg

Canada
Alzheimer Society of Canada
20 Eglinton Avenue, W., Suite 1600
Toronto, Ontario M4R 1K8
Canada
Tel: +1 416 488 8772
Helpline: 1800 616 8816
Fax: +1 416 488 3778
Email: info@alzheimer.ca
Web: www.alzheimer.ca

Chile
Corporación Alzheimer Chile
Desiderio Lemus 0143
(alt 1400 Av.Peru)
Recoleta
Santiago, Chile
Tel: +56 2 7321 532
Fax: +56 2 777 7431
Email: alzchile@adsl.tie.cl
Web: www.corporacionalzheimer.cl

China
Alzheimer's Disease Chinese
Department of Neurology
First Hospital Peking University
Beijing 100034
PR China
Tel: +8610 6521 2012

Fax: +8610 6521 2386
Email: wyhbdyy@gmail.com

Colombia
Asociacion Colombiana de Alzheimer y Desordenes Relacionados
Calle 69 A No. 10-16
Sante Fe de Bogota D.C.
Colombia
Tel/Fax: +57 1 521 9401
Email: alzheimercolombia@hotmail.com

Costa Rica
Asociación Costarricense de Alzheimer y otras Demencias Asociadas
991-2070, Sabanilla de Montes de Oca
San José 11502 2070
Costa Rica
Tel: +905 285 3919
Email: ascada.alzcr@gmail.com
Web: ascadacr.wordpress.com

Croatia
Alzheimer Disease Societies Croatia
Vlaska 24a
HR-10000 Zagreb
Croatia
Tel/Fax: +385 1560 1500
Email: alzheimer@alzheimer.hr
Web: www.alzheimer.hr

Cuba

Sección Cubana de la Enfermedad de Alzheimer
Policlinico Docente Playa
Proyecto Alzheimer, Avenida 68 # 29B y 29F
Playa Ciudad de la Habana, C.P. 11400
Cuba
Tel: +537 220 974
Fax: +537 336 857
Email: mguerra@infomed.sld.cu
Web: www.scual.sld.cu

Curaçao

Stichting Alzheimer Curaçao
Roodeweg 111
Willemstad
Curaçao
Tel: +5 999 462 3900
Fax: +5 999 462 8554
Email: alzheimer-curacao@hotmail.com

Cyprus

Pancyprian Association of Alzheimer's Disease
Stylianou Lena 47, Flat 1
6021 Larnaca
Cyprus
Tel: +357 24 627 104
Fax: +357 24 627 106
Email: alzhcyprus@cytanet.com.cy

Czech Republic
eská alzheimerovská spole nost
Centre of Gerontology
Simunkova 1600
18200 Praha 8
Czech Republic
Tel: +420 286 883 676
Fax: +420 286 882 788
Email: martina.matlova@gerontocentrum.cz
Web: www.alzheimer.cz

Denmark
Alzheimerforeningen
Ny Kongensgade 20, st.tv.
1557 Copenhagen V
Denmark
Tel: +45 39 40 04 88
Fax: +45 39 61 66 69
Email: post@alzheimer.dk
Web: www.alzheimer.dk

Dominican Republic
Asociacion Dominicana de Alzheimer
Apartado Postal # 3321
Santo Domingo
Republica Dominicana
Tel: +1 809 544 1711
Fax: +1 809 544 1731
Email: asocalzheimer@codetel.net.do

Ecuador *
Fundacion Alzheimer Ecuador
Centro Medico Pasteur
Ave. Eloy Alfaro e Italia
2do Piso. Consultorio 204
Quito
Ecuador
Tel: +593 2 2521 660
Fax: +593 2 2594 997
Email: gmatute@uio.satnet.net

Egypt
Egyptian Alzheimer Group
c/o Professor A Ashour
233 26 July Street
Giza 12411
Cairo
Egypt
Tel: +202 334 70 133
Fax: +202 330 23 270
Email: ashourabdelmoneim@yahoo.com

El Salvador
Asociacion de Familiares Alzheimer de El Salvador
Sara Zaldivar,
Colonia Costa Rica, Avenida Irazu
San Salvador
El Salvador   Tel: +503 2237 0787
Email: jrlopezcontreras@yahoo.com

Ethiopia *
Ye Ethiopia Alzhiemers Beshitegnoch Mahber
P. O. Box 28657/1000
Addis Ababa
Ethiopia
Tel: +251 91 113 8547
Email: ninates2002@yahoo.com

Finland
Alzheimer Society of Finland
Luotsikatu 4E
00160 Helsinki
Finland
Tel: +358 9 6226 2010
Fax: +358 9 6226 2020
Email: anna.tamminen@muistiliitto.fi
Web: www.muistiliitto.fi

France
Association France Alzheimer
21 Boulevard Montmartre
75002 Paris
France
Tel: +33 1 42 97 52 41
Fax: +33 1 42 96 04 70
Email: contact@francealzheimer.org
Web: www.francealzheimer.org

Germany
Deutsche Alzheimer Gesellschaft
Friedrichstr. 236
10969 Berlin
Germany
Tel: +49 30 315 057 33
Helpline: 01803 171 017
Fax: +49 30 315 057 35
Email: deutsche.alzheimer.ges@t-online.de
Web: www.deutsche-alzheimer.de

Gibraltar *
The Gibraltar Alzheimer's and Dementia Support Group
P.O. Box 1196
Gibraltar
Tel: +350 2007 1049
Email: gadsg@gibtelecom.net

Greece
Greek Association of AD and Related Disorders
Petrou Sindika 13
Thessaloniki
Hellas
Greece
Tel/Fax : +30 2310 810 411
Helpline: +30 2310 909 000
Email: info@alzheimer-hellas.gr
Web: www.alzheimer-hellas.gr

Guatemala
Asociación ERMITA, Alzheimer de Guatemala
10a. Calle 11-63
Zona 1, Ave. 1-48 Zona 1
Apto B, P O Box 2978
01901 Guatemala
Tel: +502 2 320 324
Fax: +502 2 381 122
Email: alzguate@quetzal.net

Honduras
Asociación Hondureña de Alzheimer
Apartado Postal 5005
Tegucigalpa
Honduras, C.A.
Tel: +504 239 4512
Fax: +504 232 4580
Email: alzheimerhn@ashalz.org
Web: www.ashalz.org

Hong Kong SAR
Hong Kong Alzheimer's Disease Association
G/F, Wang Yip House
Wang Tau Hom Estate
Kowloon, Hong Kong SAR
China
Tel: +852 23 381 120
Carer Hotline: +852 23 382 277
Fax: +852 23 38 0772

Email: headoffice@hkada.org.hk
Web: www.hkada.org.hk

Hungary
Hungarian Alzheimer Society
Csaba u. 7A
H-1122
Budapest 1122
Hungary
Tel:+36 1 214 1022
Fax: +36 1 214 1022
Email: ehimmer@t-online.hu
Web: www.alzheimerweb.hu

Iceland *
FAAS
Austurburn 31
104 Reyjkjavik
Iceland
Tel: +354 533 1088
Fax: +354 533 1086
Email: faas@alzheimer.is
Web: www.alzheimer.is

India
Alzheimer's & Related Disorders Society of India
Guruvayoor Road
PO Box 53 Kunnamkulam
Kerala 680 503

India
Tel: +91 4885 223 801
Fax: +91 4885 224 817
Email: ardsinationaloffice@gmail.com or alzheimr@md2.vsnl.net.in
Web: www.alzheimer.org.in

Indonesia
IAzA Secretariat
jl. Nanas 3
no 28 Utan Kayu Selatan
Jakarta
Timur 13120
Indonesia
Tel: +62 21 174 05486
Fax: +62 21 174 05482
Email: martina_wiwie@yahoo.com

Iran
Iran Alzheimer Association
Shahrak Ekbatan
North Sattari Exit
Next to Bassij Building
Tehran 13969
Iran
Tel: +98 21 4651 122
Fax: +98 21 4651 122
Email: info@alzheimer.ir
Web: www.alzheimer.ir

Ireland
Alzheimer Society of Ireland
National Office
Temple Road
Blackrock, Co. Dublin
Ireland
Tel: +353 1 284 6616
Helpline: +353 1 800 341 341
Fax: +353 1 284 6030
Email: info@alzheimer.ie
Web: www.alzheimer.ie

Israel
Alzheimer's Association of Israel
P O Box 8261
Ramat Gan
Israel 52181
Tel: +972 3 578 7660
Fax: +972 3 578 7661
Email: office@alz-emda.org.il
Web: www.alz-il.net

Italy
Federazione Alzheimer Italia
Via Tommaso Marino 7
20121 Milano
Italy
Tel: +39 02 809 767
Fax: +39 02 875 781

Email: alzit@tin.it
Web: www.alzheimer.it

Jamaica
Alzheimer's Jamaica
52 Duke Street
Kingston
Jamaica
Tel: +1 876 927 8967
Fax: +1 876 927 6155
Email: alzheimerja@cwjamaica.com

Japan
Alzheimer's Association Japan
c/o Kyoto Social Welfare Hall
Horikawa-Marutamachi, Kamigyo-Ku
Kyoto
Japan 602-8143
Tel: +81 75 811 8195
Fax: +81 75 811 8188
Email: office@alzheimer.or.jp
Web: www.alzheimer.or.jp

Jordan *
Jordanian Alzheimer Association
Faculty of Medicine
University of Jordan
P.O. Box 13490
Amman 11942

Jordan
Tel: +96 279 659 6390 or +96 265 355 000
Fax: +96 265 356 746
Email: e.alkhateeb@ju.edu.jo

Kenya *
Alzheimer's Association of Kenya
University of Nairobi
AIC Building, Flat No. 4
Ralph Bunche Road
P.O. Box 48423-00100
Nairobi
Kenya
Tel: +254 0202 716 315
Fax: +254 0202 717 168
Email: dmndetei@uonbi.ac.ke

Lebanon
Alzheimer's Association Lebanon
Chammah Building, 7th floor - Facing Mikado
Monot Street
Achrafieh
Lebanon
Tel: +961 3 245 606
Email: d.mansour@alzlebanon.org
Web: www.alzlebanon.org

Luxembourg *
Association Luxembourg Alzheimer
BP 5021
L-1050
Luxembourg
Tel: +352 42 16 76 1
Fax: +352 42 16 76 30
Helpline: +352 26 432 432
Email: info@alzheimer.lu
Web: www.alzheimer.lu

Macau SAR *
Macau Alzheimer's Disease Association
9/F, Macau Landmark
555 Avenida da Amizade
Macau SAR
China
Fax: +853 8295 6225 or +853 2878 2233
Fax: +853 2836 5204 or +853 2878 1218
Email: info@mada.org.mo
Web: www.mada.org.mo

Macedonia
Association of Alzheimer Disease - Skopje Macedonia
Ul. 50 Divizija br 34
Ordinacija Pasoski
1000 Skopje
Macedonia

Tel: +389 7576 1025 or +389 2317 9805
Email: makalzheimer@yahoo.com

Madagascar *
Madagascar Alzheimer Association
Masoandro Mody
Lot VK 70 Bis A
Fenomanana Mahazoarivo
BP 3081 - 101 Antananarivo
Madagascar
Tel: +26 120 226 1202
Email: muriel.rason.andriamaro@moov.mg
Web: www.madagascar-alzheimer.org

Malaysia
Alzheimer's Disease Foundation Malaysia
No. 6 Lorong 11/8E, Sec. 11
46200 Petaling Jaya
Selangor Darul Ehsan
Malaysia
Tel: +603 7956 2008 or +603 7958 3008
Fax: +603 7960 8482
Email: office.adfm@gmail.com
Web: www.adfm.org.my

Malta
Malta Dementia Society
Room 135
Department of Pharmacy

University of Malta
Msida
Malta
Email: info@maltadementiasociety.org.mt
Web: www.maltadementiasociety.org.mt

Mauritius
Alzheimer Association Mauritius
Old Moka Rd
Belle Rose
Quatre Bornes
Mauritius
Tel: +230 466 0731
Helpline +230 800 1111
Email: assocalzheimer@intnet.mu
Web: http://mauritiusalzheimer.intnet.mu

Mexico
Federación Mexicana de Alzheimer
Av. Manrique 540
Colinas de San Gerardo
Tampico, Tamaulipas 89367
Mexico
Tel: +52 81 8333 6713 or +52 81 8347 4072
Helpline: 01 800 00 33362
Email: alzheimerfedma@yahoo.com
Web: http://fedma.org.mx/

Monaco*
AMPA
Europa Résidence
Place des Moulins
98000 Monaco
Monaco
Tel: +377 92 16 58 88
Fax: +377 92 16 58 81
Email: info@ampa-monaco.com
Web: www.ampa-monaco.com

Namibia *
Elzabeth Swart (support groups)
Tel/Fax: + 264 61 227 023
Email: jtpot@mweb.com.na

Nepal *
Alzheimer's Association Nepal
P.O. Box 4795
20200 Kathmandu
Nepal
Tel: +977 1557 0361 or +977 1557 4380
Fax: +977 1 446 3029
Email: alz.nepal@gmail.com

Netherlands
Alzheimer Nederland
Post Bus 183
3980 CD BUNNIK

The Netherlands
Tel: +31 30 659 6900
Helpline: 030 656 7511
Fax: +31 30 659 6901
Email: info@alzheimer-nederland.nl
Web: www.alzheimer-nederland.nl

New Zealand
Alzheimers New Zealand
Level 3, Adelphi Finance House
15 Courtenay Place
PO Box 3643
Wellington
New Zealand
Tel: +64 4 381 2362
Helpline: 0800 004 001
Fax: +64 4 381 2365
Email: nationaloffice@alzheimers.org.nz
Web: www.alzheimers.org.nz

Nigeria
Alzheimer's Disease Association of Nigeria
c/o Dept. of Psychiatry
Nnamdi Azikiwe University Teaching Hospital
Nnewi Anambra State
Nigeria
Tel: +234 46 463 663
Fax: +234 46 462 496
Email: alzheimernigeria@yahoo.com

Norway *
Nasjonalforeningen Demensforbundet
Oscarsgt 36 A, Postboks
7139 Majorstua
N 0307 Oslo
Norway
Tel: +47 23 12 00 00
Helpline: +47 815 33 032
Fax: +47 23 12 00 01
Email: post@nasjonalforeningen.no
Web: www.nasjonalforeningen.no

Pakistan
Alzheimer's Pakistan
146/1 Shadman Jail Road
Lahore 54000
Pakistan
Tel: +92 42 759 6589
Fax: +92 42 757 3911
Email: info@alz.org.pk
Web: www.alz.org.pk

Panama
AFA PADEA
Via Fernandez de Córdoba, Edificio Julimar, Primer Piso, Oficina #3
Apartado Postal 6-6839
El Dorado
Panama
Email: afapadea@gmail.com

Peru

Asociacion Peruana de Enfermedad de Alzheimer y Otras Demencias
Calle Inquisicion No 135, 2do piso
Esquina Av. Caminos del Inca
Santiago de Surco
Lima 33
Peru
Tel: +511 279 2331

Philippines

Alzheimer's Disease Association of the Philippines
St Luke's Medical Center
Medical Arts Bldg, Rm 410
E Rodriguez Sr Avenue, Quezon City
Philippines
Tel/fax: +632 723 1039
Email: info@alzphilippines.com
Web: www.alzphilippines.com

Poland

Polish Alzheimer's Association
ul.E.Plater 47
00-118 Warsaw
Poland
Tel/Fax: + 48 22 622 11 22
Email: alzheimer_pl@hotmail.com
Web: www.alzheimer.pl

Portugal *
Associação Portuguesa de Familiares e Amigos de Doentes de Alzheimer
Avenida de Ceuta Norte
Lote 1 - Lojas 1 e 2 - Quinta do Loureiro
1350-410 Lisboa
Portugal
Tel: +351 21 361 0460
Fax: +351 21 361 0469
Email: geral@alzheimerportugal.org
Web: www.alzheimerportugal.org

Puerto Rico
Asociación de Alzheimer y Desórdenes Relacionados de Puerto Rico
Apartado 362026
San Juan
Puerto Rico 00936-2026
Tel: +1 787 727 4151
Fax: +1 787 727 4890
Email: alzheimerpr@alzheimerpr.org
Web: www.alzheimerpr.org

Romania
Romanian Alzheimer Society
52 Austrului Street
2nd District
024074 Bucharest
Romania
Tel: +402 1 334 8940

Fax: +402 1 334 8940
Email: contact@alz.ro
Web: www.alz.ro

Russia
Association for Support of Alzheimer's Disease Victims
34 Kashirskoye shosse
115522 Moscow
Russia
Tel: +7 095 324 9615
Fax: +7 095 114 4925
Email: sigavrilova@yandex.ru
Web: www.alzrus.org

Scotland
Alzheimer Scotland - Action on Dementia
22 Drumsheugh Gardens
Edinburgh EH3 7RN
Scotland
Tel: +44 131 243 1453
Helpline: 0808 808 3000
Fax: +44 131 243 1450
Email: alzheimer@alzscot.org
Web: www.alzscot.org

Serbia *
Alzheimer Society of Serbia and Montenegro
Dr Subotica 6
Institute of Neurology

Belgrade 11000
Serbia
Tel: +381 11 361 4122
Fax: +381 11 684 577
Email: dpavlovic@drenik.net

Singapore
Alzheimer's Disease Association
Blk 157 Lorong 1 Toa Payoh
#01-1195
Singapore 310157
Tel: +65 6353 8734
Singapore 310157
Tel: +65 6353 8734
Fax: +65 6353 8518
Email: adahq@alz.org.sg
Web: www.alz.org.sg

Sint Maarten
Sint Maarten Alzheimer Foundation
St Petersroad 65
St Peters
Sint Maarten
Tel: + 599 520 0777
Email: alzheimersxm@gmail.com

Slovak Republic
Slovak Alzheimer's Society
Mlynarovicova 21

851 03 Bratislava
Slovak Republic
Tel: +421 7 594 13 353
Fax: +421 7 547 74 276
Email: nilunova@savba.sk
Web: www.alzheimer.sk

South Africa
Alzheimer's South Africa
10 Boskruin Business Park
Bosbok Road
Randpark Ridge ext 58
2169
South Africa
Tel: +27 11 792 2511/8387
Fax: +27 11 792 7135
Helpline: 0860 102 681 (Mornings from 09h00)
Email: info@alzheimers.org.za
Web: www.alzheimers.org.za

South Korea
Alzheimer's Association, Korea
#52, Machon 2-Dong
Songpa-ku
Seoul 138-122
South Korea
Tel: +82 2 431 9963
Helpline: +82 2 431 9993
Fax: +82 2 431 9964

Email: afcde01@unitel.co.kr
Web: www.alzza.or.kr

Spain
Confederación Española de Familiares de Enfermos de Alzheimer
C/ Pedro Miguel Alcatarena nº 3
31014 Pamplona (Navarra)
Spain
Tel: +34 902 174 517
Fax: +34 948 265 739
Email: ceafa@ceafa.es
Web: www.ceafa.es

Sri Lanka
Lanka Alzheimer's Foundation
110 Ketawalamulla Lane
Colombo 10
Sri Lanka
Helpline + 94 11 2667080
General Lines + 94 11 266 7082 or +94 11 266 7084
Fax: +94 11 266 7087
Email: alzheimers@alzlanka.org
Web: www.alzlanka.org

Suriname *
Surinam Alzheimer Society (SAS)
Papajastraat 30
Paramaribo
Suriname

Tel: +597 0859 0527
Email: dennisrust@sr.net

Sweden
Alzheimerföreningen i Sverige
Karl XII gatan 1
221 00 Lund
Sweden
Tel: +46 46 14 73 18
Fax: +46 46 18 89 76
Email: info@alzheimerforeningen.se
Web: www.alzheimerforeningen.se

Switzerland
Association Alzheimer Suisse
8 Rue des Pêcheurs
CH-1400 Yverdon-les-Bains
Switzerland
Tel: +41 24 426 2000
Fax: +41 24 426 2167
Email: alz@bluewin.ch
Web: www.alz.ch

Syria
Syrian Alzheimer and Memory Diseases Society
PO Box 14189
Damascus
Syria
Tel: +963 94 74 1955

Fax: +963 11 54 21893
Email: syria@icbl.org

TADA Chinese Taipei
TADA
10F-1, No. 206, Sec. 2
Nanchang Road
100
Taipei
100
Taipei
Taiwan
Tel: +886 2 23 149 690
Fax: +886 2 23 147 508
Email: tada.tada@msa.hinet.net
Web: www.tada2002.org.tw

Thailand
Alzheimer's and Related Disorders Association of Thailand
114 Pinakorn 4
Boramratchachunee Road
Talingchan
Bangkok 10170
Thailand
Tel: +66 2 880 8542/7539
Fax: +66 2 880 7244
Email: chansirikarn.c@gmail.com
Web: www.azthai.org

Trinidad and Tobago
Alzheimer's Association of Trinidad and Tobago
c/o Soroptimist International Port of Spain
15 Nepaul Street
St James, Port of Spain
Republic of Trinidad and Tobago
Tel: +1 868 622 6134
Fax: +1 868 627 6731
Email: nebinniss@gmail.com

Tunisia *
Association Alzheimer Tunisie
BP N°116
Cité Elkhadra
1003 Tunis
Tunisia
Tel: +216 98 613 976
Fax: +216 98 704 592
Email: alzheimer.tunisie@gmail.com

Turkey
Turkish Alzheimer Association
Halaskargazi Cad. No: 115 Da: 4 Harbiye
Istanbul
Turkey
Tel: +90 212 224 41 89   Helpline: 0800 211 8024
Fax: +90 212 296 05 79
Email: alzdernek@alzheimerdernegi.org.tr
Web: www.alzheimerdernegi.org.tr

Ukraine *
The Association for the Problems of Alzheimer's Disease
Institute of Gerontology
67 Vyshgorodskaya Street
04114 Kiev
Ukraine
Tel: +380 44 431 0526
Fax: +380 44 432 9956

United Kingdom (except Scotland)
Alzheimer's Society
Devon House
58 St Katharine's Way
London E1W 1JX
United Kingdom
Tel: +44 20 7423 3500
Helpline: 0845 300 0336
Fax: +44 20 7423 3501
Email: enquiries@alzheimers.org.uk
Web: www.alzheimers.org.uk

United States of America
Alzheimer's Association
225 N Michigan Avenue
Suite 1700
Chicago, Illinois 60601-7633
United States of America
Tel: +1 312 335 8700
Helpline: 1 800 272 3900

Fax: +1 866 699 1246
Email: info@alz.org
Web: www.alz.org

Uruguay
Asociación Uruguaya de Alzheimer y Similares
Magallanes 1320
11200 Montevideo
Uruguay
Tel: +598 2 400 8797
Fax: +598 2 400 8797
Email: audasur@gmail.com
Web: http://audas.wordpress.com

Venezuela
Fundación Alzheimer de Venezuela
Calle El Limon, Qta Mi Muñe, El Cafetal
Caracas
Venezuela
Tel: +58 212 414 6129
Fax: +58 212 9859 183
Email: alzven@gmail.com
Web: www.alzheimer.org.ve

Zimbabwe
Zimbabwe Alzheimer's and Related Disorders Association
PO Box CH 832
Chisipite
Harare

Zimbabwe
Tel: +263 779 714 905 or +263 449 4409
Fax: +263 470 4487
Email: zarda@zol.co.zw

Regional groups
Europe
Alzheimer Europe
145 route de Thionville
L-2611
Luxembourg
Tel: +352 29 79 70
Fax: +352 29 79 72
Email: info@alzheimer-europe.org
Web: www.alzheimer-europe.org

Latin America
Alzheimer Iberoamerica
C/ Pedro Alcatarena nº 3 Bajo
31014 Pamplona (Navarra)
Spain
Tel: +34 902 174 517
Fax: +34 948 265 739
Email: ceafa@ceafa.es
Web: http://alzheimeriberoamerica.org/

AIDS Dementia
Global AIDS Foundation Headquarters
The Netherlands
Keizersgracht 518
1017 EK AmsterdamKeizersgracht 518
1017 EK Amsterdam
THE NETHERLANDS
Tel. +31 (0)20 626 6267
global.info@aidshealth.org

Asia Pacific Bureau
S7 Panchsheel Park
110017 New Delhi, INDIA
Tel. +91 11 417 455 41/42

East-West Africa Bureau
Plot 13, Nakasero Road
P.O. Box 22914
Kampala, UGANDA
Tel. +256 414 346 311

Latin America Bureau
Gaspar Bolaños #648
Jardines Alcalde
Guadalajara, Jalisco, MEXICO 44290
Tel. +1 213 361 2524

Southern Africa Bureau
Shop 9, Umlazi Mall, W. Section

Umlazi, Durban, SOUTH AFRICA
Tel. +27 31 906 0452
Tel. +31 (0)20 626 6267
global.info@aidshealth.org

Asia Pacific Bureau
S7 Panchsheel Park
110017 New Delhi, INDIA
Tel. +91 11 417 455 41/42

East-West Africa Bureau
Plot 13, Nakasero Road
P.O. Box 22914
Kampala, UGANDA
Tel. +256 414 346 311

Latin America Bureau
Gaspar Bolaños #648
Jardines Alcalde
Guadalajara, Jalisco, MEXICO 44290
Tel. +1 213 361 2524

Southern Africa Bureau
Shop 9, Umlazi Mall, W. Section
Umlazi, Durban, SOUTH AFRICA
Tel. +27 31 906 0452

United States Headquarters
AIDS Healthcare Foundation
6255 W. Sunset Blvd 21st Fl.
Los Angeles, CA 90028
United States
Tel. (323) 860-5200

amfAR New York
120 Wall Street, 13th Floor
New York, NY 10005-3908
Tel. (212) 806-1600
amfAR Washington D.C.
1150 17th Street, NW, Suite 406
Washington, DC 20036-4622
Tel. (202) 331-8600

Elton John AIDS Foundation
USA:
584 Broadway, Suite 906
New York, NY 10012
UK:
1 Blythe Road
London, W14 OHG
United Kingdom
Telephone: +44 (0) 20 7603 9996

Chemo Brain
Chemobraininfo.org
25A Cresent Drive, Suite 345

Pleasant Hill, CA 94523
Telephone: 925-262-4250
Website: www.Chemobraininfo.org

Open-Heart Surgery Brain-Related Changes
Best Resource I can locate for this issue:
Miller Family Heart & Vascular Institute
Cleveland Clinic Organization
Resource & Information Contact
Telephone: 216-445-9288
Toll Free Number: 866-289-6911

Traumatic Brain Injury
Brain Injury Association of Canada
Phone: 866-977-2492
Founded in 2003, the Brain Injury Association of Canada (BIAC)'s mission is to improve the quality of life for all Canadians affected by acquired brain injury, and promote brain injury prevention. BIAC partners with national, provincial/territorial and regional associations, and other stakeholders to facilitate post-trauma research, education and advocacy. BIAC is incorporated as a national charitable organization under the Canada Corporations Act and Canada Revenue Agency.

Brain Injury Australia
Phone: 02 9591 1094
Founded in 1986, Brain Injury Australia (BIA) represents all Australians with acquired brain injury. BIA represents, through its State and Territory Member Organizations, the needs of people with an acquired brain injury, their families and caregivers. BIA operates at a

national level to ensure that all people living with acquired brain injury have access to the supports and resources they need.

Brain Injury New Zealand
Phone: 09 414 5693

Brain Injury New Zealand (BIANZ) represents the regional Brain Injury Associations around New Zealand. These regional associations provide education, advocacy, support and information to any person with a brain injury and their families and/or caregivers. The national office provides support for the regional associations, national level advocacy, and political review.

European Brain Injury Society
Phone: +32 (0)2 522 20 03

EBIS is a European association that serves traumatic brain injured persons and victims of acquired cerebral lesions: stroke, anoxia, encephalitis, brain tumor. EBIS members have access to a network of brain injury professionals and services. Other benefits include seminars, workshops and advice about relevant activities of the European Union. EBIS has 165 individual and institutional members from all the countries of the European Union, plus Switzerland.

Headway UK
Phone: 0808 800 2244

Headway is a charity set up to give help and support to people affected by brain injury. It does this both locally and nationally. Headway's mission is to promote understanding of all aspects of brain injury and to provide information, support and services to people with a brain injury, their families and carers.

International Brain Injury Association
Phone: 703-960-0027
Founded in 1993, the International Brain Injury Association (IBIA) is dedicated to the development and support of multidisciplinary medical and clinical professionals, advocates, policy makers, consumers and others who work to improve outcomes and opportunities for persons with brain injury.

TBI Hormone Imbalance Syndrome
Millenneum Medical Centers, Mark L. Gordon MD, Director
16661 Ventura Blvd. Suite 716
Encino, CA 91436 USA
Telephone: 818-990-1166
Website: https//www.tbimedlegal.com

Brain Injury Association of America
1608 Spring Hill Road, Suite 110
Vienna, VA 22182
Telephone: 703-761-0750
National Brain Injury Information Center: 1-800-444—6443

Chronic Traumatic Encephalopathy (CTE)
Center for the Study of Chronic Traumatic Encephalopathy
Boston University, Boston, Massachusetts
For all general inquiries:
cste@bu.edu
For research matters:
Christine Baugh
Research Coordinator

(617) 638-6143
cbaugh@bu.edu
For urgent brain donation matters, page CSTE staff at:
Primary: (617) 638-5795 pager ID# 6144
Secondary: (508) 322-0875

Sports Legacy Institute
P.O. Box 181225
Boston, MA 02118
Telephone: 781-262-3324
Email: info@sportslegacy.org

Fronto-Temporal Lobe Dementia
Association for Frontotemporal Lobe Degeneration
Radnor Station Building 2, Suite 320
Radnor, Pennsylvania 19087
Telephone : 267-514-7221
Toll Free Helpline: 866-507-7222

Huntington's Disease
Huntington's Disease Society of America
505 Eighth Avenue, Suite 902
New York, NY 10018
Telephone: 212-242-1968
Toll Free: 1-800-345-4372

Parkinson's Disease
National Parkinson Foundation, Inc.
1501 N.W. 9th Avenue, Bob Hope Road

Miami, Florida 33136
Telephone 305-243-6666; Toll Free: 1-800-327-4545
Toll Free Helpline: 1-800-473-4636
Email: contact@parkinson.org

The Michael J. Fox Foundation for Parkinson's Research
Grand Central Station
P.O. Box 4777
New York, NY 10163-4777
Telephone: 1-800-708-7644
Website: www.michaeljfox.org

Lewy Bodies Dementia
Lewy Body Dementia Association
912 Killian Hill Road, S.W.
Lilburn, GA 30047
Caregiver Toll Free Helpline: 1-800-539-9767
Website: www.lbda.org

Vascular Dementia
World Stroke Organization
WSO Administrative Offices
Maria Grupper
Liaison Officer
1-3, rue de Chantepoulet
CH-1211 Geneva
Switzerland
Email: admin@world-stroke.org
www.world-stroke.org

National Institute of Neurological Disorders & Stroke
P.O. Box 5801
Bethesda, MD 20824
Telephone: 1-800-352-9424
Website: www.ninds.nih.gov

National Stroke Association
9707 East Easter Lane, Suite B
Centinnial, CO 80112-
Telephone: 303-649-9299
Toll Free: 1-800-787-6537
Website: www.stroke.org

Caregiver Support
Family Caregiver Alliance
785 Market St, Suite 750
San Francisco, CA 94103
Telephone: 415-434-3388
Toll Free: 1-800-445-8106
Website: www.caregiver.org

National Family Caregivers Association
10400 Connecticut Avenue, Suite 500
Kensington, MD 20895-3944
Telephone: 301-942-6430
Toll Free: 1-800-896-3650
Website: www.nfcacares.org